Fantastically Free

The Savvy Mom's Guide to Living a Safe, Happy, and Healthy Life with Food Allergies

TIFFANY DESILVA, MSW, CPC, CHC

Dedication

This book is dedicated to my three daughters.

You each inspire me to live fantastically free every day.

Your zest for life is contagious, your resilience is unfailing,
and your strength is beyond measure.

You are my heart and my heroes.

Fantastically Free: The Savvy Mom's Guide to Living a Safe, Happy, and Healthy Life with Food Allergies

To contact the publisher, visit
www.BrightFireLiving.com

To contact the author, visit
www.FantasticallyFree.com

ISBN-13: 978-0-9961728-0-6
ISBN-10: 0996172807

Printed in the United States of America

TABLE OF CONTENTS

Acknowledgements

Thank you to my husband, Brad, and my three daughters for supporting me and encouraging through the journey of writing this book. I would not have been able to do it without you!

Thank you to my friend, Trudy Scott, for first inspiring me to write this book and helping me to see all of its possibilities.

Many thanks to Joshua Rosenthal, of the Institute for Integrative Nutrition, for helping me to realize the enormous need for this book and encouraging me to share my message with the world.

Thank you to Lindsey Smith for walking with me through the book writing process and cheering me on along the way.

Thank you to my accountability partners, Sheila Sekuterski and Rachel Abbett for helping me to finish the book, no matter what.

Introduction

As the mother of three beautiful and brilliant girls with multiple food allergies, I know just how challenging managing food allergies can be. I also know that having food allergies doesn't have to stop you from living an amazing life or keep you from enjoying the people and things that matter most to you.

I've been managing food allergies for over a decade now. Each of my daughters were diagnosed with their first food allergy (cow's milk) when they were just infants. Although I nursed each one, they reacted to the dairy that I consumed. Luckily, they have all outgrown their dairy allergy but they still have many more.

In all, my children are allergic to peanut, tree nuts, egg, soy, sesame, mustard, banana, tomato, pineapple, potato, shellfish, green pea and green bean.

In addition to food allergies, we also manage autoimmune disorders, eczema, asthma, cold-induced urticaria, and environmental allergies including: ragweed, grass, tree pollen, dust, mold, cat, rabbit, and guinea pig.

As you can see, we are quite the atopic bunch. While there are a lot of things we can't eat or be around, there is an abundance of foods that we can eat and so many wonderful things that we enjoy doing.

We do NOT let food allergies put limitations on our life and you don't have to either.

This book is intended for mothers of children who are newly-diagnosed with an IgE-mediated food allergy as well as mothers who may have managed food allergies for awhile but would like to expand their knowledge base and improve their family's quality of life.

As a mother of children with food allergies, a social worker, a health and wellness coach, and lifestyle coach, my mission is to help other families live safe, healthy, and happy lives despite food allergies; this is what I call living Fantastically Free!

Think of this book as a quick start guide to get you on the path towards living your best life with food allergies. The book is divided into the 3 pillars of living Fantastically Free, Living Safely, Living Happily, and Healthy Living. Each chapter covers a different aspect of the 3 pillars. At the end of each chapter you will find quick exercises, which I call Fantastically Free Exercises. These exercises are designed to get you to take action towards actually living Fantastically Free.

Some of this information may be new to you and some of it may not be. That is completely okay. Use the information that resonates with you. You can also use the book to facilitate conversations with your child's doctor. Please remember to consult your child's doctor or another healthcare professional before making any changes to your child's care or emergency allergy plan.

Congratulations on beginning this book. Your journey towards living *Fantastically Free* is underway!

PART I:

Living Safely

Chapter 1

LEARN ALL YOU CAN ABOUT FOOD ALLERGIES

Effectively managing food allergies and living well with them requires a commitment to learning everything you can about them and keeping your knowledge base fresh, accurate, and up-to-date. Food allergy is a relatively new field of study and information, best practices, and guidelines change quickly.

THE DEFINITION OF FOOD ALLERGY

Before we can begin to discuss how to live a safe, happy, and healthy life with food allergies, we need to define what a food allergy is. There is a lot of confusion around the term "food allergy." Unfortunately, many people mistakenly use the terms food allergy, sensitivity, and intolerance interchangeably.

If fact, while approximately 20% of the US population reports altering their diet due to adverse reactions to food, it is believed that only approximately 6% of children and 3% to 4% of adults actually have a food allergy.[1] This discrepancy is due to the fact that people tend to categorize any adverse food reaction as an allergy.

Also, the phrase "food sensitivity" is a broad umbrella term commonly used to refer to any adverse reaction to food, including, but not limited to food allergy and food intolerance.

Food intolerance is a non-immunologic adverse reaction caused by an inability to digest a particular food due to an enzyme deficiency. A common example of this is lactose intolerance.

The inability to digest lactose in milk and dairy products leads to the production of excess fluid in the gastrointestinal tract which results in cramping or abdominal pain and diarrhea.[2] While uncomfortable to deal with, lactose intolerance is not life-threatening. In fact, many times you can still consume dairy products or milk without any symptoms if they are lactose free or if you consume them with the enzyme lactase. In contrast, if you have an allergy to milk protein, even a small amount can trigger a dangerously severe reaction.

A food allergy is an adverse immune response triggered by food protein.[3] When I use the term "food allergy" in this book, I am specifically referring to IgE-mediated food allergies.

Immunoglobulin E (IgE) antibodies, believed to fight off parasites and intestinal worms, play a significant role in most allergic diseases, including asthma, angioedema, hay fever, hives, and anaphylaxis.[4]

IgE-mediated food allergies occur when your immune system makes specific immunoglobulin E antibodies to certain food allergens.[5] These IgE antibodies float through your blood stream and attach to mast cells and basophils. Mast cells are immune cells that reside in your body's tissues, especially in your nose, throat, lungs, gastrointestinal tract and skin. Basophils are white blood cells. Both mast cells and basophils contain histamine.

When someone with an IgE-mediated food allergy is exposed to a food allergen, usually through ingestion, the allergen binds to the IgE antibodies that are attached to mast cells and basophils. This causes the mast cells and basophils to release large amounts of chemicals, including histamine.

These chemicals trigger the various symptoms of an allergic reaction, depending on the tissue in which they are released. The symptoms can range from a mild reaction to a severe, life-threatening, systemic allergic reaction called anaphylaxis.[6]

SYMPTOMS OF AN ALLERGIC REACTION

The first symptoms of an allergic reaction may include itching, burning, or irritation of the lips, mouth, or throat. As the food enters the digestive tract, you may notice nausea, vomiting, abdominal pain and diarrhea. Feeling unwell, anxious, itchy, faint, confused, and congested is possible as the allergen enters the circulatory system. 80 to 90% of patients report some sort of skin reactions, including hives, itching, and swelling.

Other symptoms include throat tightening, hoarseness, difficulty breathing, and chest tightness. In some cases, these symptoms may be quickly followed by a loss of consciousness and death may occur from suffocation (due to swelling of the throat) or from shock and cardiac arrhythmia. Death may occur within only a few minutes of ingesting an allergen.[7] People with asthma are at increased risk of severe reactions.

It's important to note that symptoms can occur in any order and not all symptoms occur in every case of anaphylaxis. You should also know that the first line treatment for anaphylaxis is epinephrine.[8] A delay in administering epinephrine is associated with increased risk of fatal allergic reactions.

CONDITIONS EVERY MOTHER OF CHILDREN WITH FOOD ALLERGIES SHOULD KNOW

Eosinophilic Esophagitis

Eosinophilic esophagitis (EoE) is characterized by eosinophilic inflammation of the esophagus. Children with EoE commonly present with feeding disorders, vomiting, reflux symptoms, and abdominal pain. Adolescents with EoE often experience difficulty swallowing and esophageal food impactions (food stuck in their throat).[9]

Food Protein-Induced Enterocolitis Syndrome

Food protein-induced enterocolitis syndrome (FPIES) is a non–IgE-mediated gastrointestinal food hypersensitivity that manifests as profuse, repetitive vomiting, often with diarrhea, leading to acute dehydration and lethargy or weight loss and failure to thrive if chronic. FPIES is elicited most commonly by milk and soy proteins; however, rice, oat, and other solid foods may also elicit FPIES.[10]

Atopic Dermatitis

Atopic Dermatitis is also referred to as atopic eczema or eczema. It is a chronic skin disease characterized by itchy, inflamed skin. Atopic dermatitis is one of the most common pediatric skin disorders and is seen in up to 10% of children. Approximately 30% of children with severe atopic dermatitis have some type of food reaction. These reactions vary from classic IgE-mediated symptoms like hives and anaphylaxis to eczema flares. Eczema flares can be immediate or delayed up to 24 hours after ingestion.[11]

Allergic Contact Dermatitis

Allergic contact dermatitis is a form of eczema caused by a cell-mediated allergic reaction. It is characterized by a red, itchy reaction where the skin has come into contact with a substance that the immune system recognizes as foreign, such as chemical haptens that are additives in foods or that may occur naturally in foods like mango, in plants like poison ivy, or certain preservatives in creams and lotions.[12]

Contact Dermatitis

Contact dermatitis is a localized reaction that includes redness, itching, and burning where the skin has come into contact with an allergen or with an irritant such as an acid, a cleaning product, or other chemical.[13]

Acute Urticaria

Acute urticaria, also known as hives, is a common symptom of IgE-mediated food allergies, though food allergy is not the only cause. Urticaria or hives are lesions that develop after ingesting a food and often appear to be round or irregular-shaped wheals that range in size from a few millimeters to several centimeters.[14]

Contact Urticaria

Contact Urticaria is divided into two subtypes: Immunological (due to IgE-mediated allergic reaction) and nonimmunological (ie. caused by direct histamine release.[15]

Nonimmunological contact urticaria is an immediate reaction not requiring prior exposure to the substance, while immunological contact urticaria is an IgE-mediated hypersensitivity reaction in which the patient's immune system has been previously sensitized to the substance.[16]

Cold Urticaria

Cold urticaria is a reaction to cold which causes your skin to develop hives. Some people may experience only minor reactions to cold, while others may have severe reactions, including anaphylaxis. Swimming in cold water is the most common cause of a systemic anaphylactic reaction which could be fatal.

Cholinergic Urticaria

Cholinergic urticaria is also known as heat urticaria. Cholinergic urticaria is a reaction to heat which causes your skin to break out in hives. Common triggers for heat urticaria include the sun, exercising, bathing in hot or warm water, spending time in a heated environment, and emotional triggers like anxiety, emotional stress, or excitement.[17]

Asthma

Asthma is a chronic lung disease that that affects people of all ages, though it typically begins during childhood. More than 25 million people are known to have asthma in the United States. Of these 25 million people, approximately 7 million are children.[18]

Common symptoms of asthma include recurring episodes of wheezing, chest tightness, shortness of breath, and coughing. It is common for coughing to occur at night or early in the morning.

Asthma causes inflammation of the airways which makes the airways swollen and very sensitive. The airways tend to react strongly to certain inhaled substances.

When the airways react, the muscles around them tighten which narrows the airways, causing less air to flow into the lungs. The swelling may also worsen, making the airways even narrower. Cells in the airways may produce more mucus which can further narrow the airways.[19]

Sometimes asthma symptoms are mild and go away on their own or after minimal treatment with asthma medicine, such as albuterol. Other times, symptoms may continue to get worse.[20]

When symptoms worsen or become more numerous, you having what is commonly known as an *asthma attack*. Asthma attacks also are called asthma flares or exacerbations.[21]

It is important to treat asthma symptoms as soon as they begin. This will help prevent symptoms from worsening and causing a severe asthma attack.

Severe asthma attacks may require emergency care, and they can be fatal.

If your child has asthma, be sure to create an asthma care plan with your physician so that you know what to do to manage asthma-related symptoms.

Allergic Rhinitis

According to the American College of Allergy, Asthma and Immunology (ACAAI), allergic rhinitis affects between 40 million and 60 million people in the United States.[22]

Allergic rhinitis, as with other allergies, develops when the body's immune system becomes sensitized and overreacts to something in the environment.

Allergic Rhinitis is commonly referred to as hay fever or respiratory allergy. You might also hear it referred to as having an environmental allergy.

Symptoms of environmental allergies include:

- ▶ Runny nose

- ▶ Nasal congestion (stuffy nose)

- ▶ Itchy eyes

- ▶ Puffy or swollen eyes

- ▶ Itchy mouth or throat

- ▶ Itchy skin

- ▶ Sneezing

- ▶ Coughing

Common environmental allergy triggers include seasonal allergens like pollen, grass, trees, and weeds, as well as perennial allergens like, dust, mold, pet hair, pet dander, and cockroaches. Other triggers include irritants such as cigarette smoke, perfume, car exhaust, air fresheners and deodorizers.

Oral Allergy Syndrome

Oral Allergy syndrome (OAS) is an IgE-mediated allergic reaction which involves only the oral mucosa. Most people describe it as itching around the mouth area. Unlike typical IgE-mediated food allergy, symptoms disappear once the food is swallowed or removed from the mouth.[23]

Oral allergy syndrome is also called pollen-food syndrome. It is caused by cross-reactivity between allergens found in pollen and in raw foods such as fruits, vegetables, nuts, and spices.[24]

Generally speaking, unlike most other food allergies, you can typically tolerate these same symptom-triggering foods if they are cooked but not if they are raw. This is because the symptom-causing proteins are altered enough by heat during the cooking process that the immune system no longer recognizes them as a threat.[25]

It is possible for people with OAS to experience anaphylaxis, a severe and even life-threatening systemic allergic reaction, so be sure to discuss your symptoms with your allergist and create an action plan, especially if your symptoms go beyond an itchy mouth.

Exercise-Induced Anaphylaxis

Exercise-Induced Anaphylaxis is a severe allergic reaction that is triggered by physical activity.

Autoimmune Disorders

An autoimmune disorder occurs when your immune systems mistakenly attacks and damages your body's own tissue. When you have an autoimmune disorder, your immune system does not distinguish between healthy tissue and antigens. As a result, your body develops antibodies, called auto-antibodies that set out to destroy its own normal tissues.

Celiac Disease

Celiac Disease is an autoimmune disease which is induced by gluten, a protein found in wheat, barley and rye. In Celiac disease, when gluten is ingested it causes the immune system to damage the villi, small finger-like projections found in the lining of the small intestine. Symptoms of celiac disease can vary widely from person to person and may include diarrhea, constipation, abdominal pain, weight loss, joint pain, brain fog, and numerous other symptoms.

Food Sensitivity

As, I mentioned previously, the term "food sensitivity" is a broad umbrella term that is used to describe any adverse reaction to food. It can be used in reference to any situation in which someone has a reproducible adverse reaction. It can be anything from getting a headache after eating a particular food to triggering an autoimmune response.

THE RISE OF FOOD ALLERGY

Allergic disease, such as eczema, asthma, allergic rhinitis, and food allergy, has reached epidemic proportions. There has been a rapid and dramatic increase in IgE-mediated food allergy In the United States (and other western countries) over the last decade. According to the CDC, food allergy increased by 50% from 1997 to 2011.[26] Non-IgE-mediated food allergies, like esosinophilic esophagitis, and autoimmune disorders like celiac disease are also on the rise.[27]

In the US, 15 million people have IgE-mediated food allergy. Of those, about 6 million are children.[28] About 39% of children surveyed had a history of severe reactions and 30% had multiple food allergies.[29]

Although there have been numerous studies undertaken to investigate the rise of both allergic disease in general and food allergy specifically, the exact cause of the epidemic is still murky. The reason that it has been so difficult to pinpoint the cause for the massive increase in food allergy is because there is no single cause but rather a number of factors contributing to the epidemic. Evidence suggests that these factors are related to our modern lifestyle.[30]

The increase in the prevalence of IgE-mediated food allergies in industrialized countries was preceded by the documented rise of other atopic or allergic conditions such as asthma, eczema, and allergic rhinitis.[31]

While the exact reason for the increase in prevalence in food allergy is unknown, the fact that it has increased in such a short period of time suggests that genetic factors alone cannot be the cause.[32]

Our genes simply do not evolve in such a short period of time. Therefore, environmental factors must play a central role in the increase of food allergy. These environmental factors affect the way our genes express themselves and influence our microbiota, both of which affect how our immunes system operates. We will discuss epigenetics and microbiome throughout this book.

As I mentioned previously, it appears that these environmental factors are linked to the *modern lifestyle.* Food allergy is more common in industrialized countries than in developing countries. In addition, migrants from developing countries acquire the same *western* risk of food allergy once they move to an industrialized country.[33]

Environmental factors, such as those associated with the hygiene hypothesis and dietary factors, have been found to play a role in the development of allergic disease.[34] Other likely factors include changes in food preparation, increase use of ant-acids and proton pump inhibitors, use of medicinal creams containing food allergens, later introduction of allergenic foods (particularly peanut) into the diet of infants.[35]

The hygiene hypothesis maintains that early exposure to diverse microbes promotes healthy immune system development and decreases the risk for developing allergies.[36] More and more research is showing that a healthy immune system reduces your risk for a number of chronic illnesses or non-communicable diseases. We will discuss this more in Part III: Healthy Living.

FANTASTICALLY FREE EXERCISE

1. Familiarize yourself with the different conditions that are associated with allergic diseases.

2. Write down any questions that you might have for your allergist.

Chapter 2

AVOID YOUR CHILD'S ALLERGENS

GETTING A DIAGNOSIS

Before you can effectively manage your child's food allergies you need to know what your child's allergens are and where they hide out. Over 15 million people have food allergies in the United States. It might surprise you to know that in the United States 90% of all allergic reactions are caused by just 8 foods. The "Top 8" food allergens, as they are called, are peanut, tree nuts, egg, cow's milk, soy, wheat, crustacean shellfish, and fish. With that being said, over 170 foods have been reported to cause IgE-mediated reactions. Anyone can be allergic to any food protein, so it is extremely important to know exactly which foods your child is allergic to in order to avoid an allergic reaction.

If you suspect that your child has a food allergy, consult a physician to confirm the diagnosis, do not rely on self-diagnosis. You may be unnecessarily excluding foods from your child's diet or worse, putting your child at risk for consuming foods that may cause a serious allergic reaction. While some people may believe that ignorance is bliss, when it comes to food allergies the risk of not knowing what your specific allergens are is too great.

Knowing what your child's allergens are truly is the first step in empowering yourself and your child in successfully managing food allergies.

If you suspect that your child may have a food allergy and are not currently under the care of an allergist, you should discuss your concerns with your primary care physician or pediatrician. He or she can make a referral to a qualified allergist.

Here are some tips for navigating the diagnosis process:

- ▶ Schedule an appointment to discuss your allergy concerns with your primary care physician or pediatrician

- ▶ Ask your doctor if your child needs to be off of any medications (ex. antihistamines, steroids) prior to your appointment, and if so, how long.

- ▶ Write down the date or dates of the suspected allergic reaction and record any symptoms your child may have experienced so that you can relate an accurate history to the doctor. The most important tool for diagnosing food allergy is an accurate clinical history.

- ▶ If you happened to have captured any photographs of hives, eczema flares, or swelling that your child might have had, take those along as well.

- ▶ Also, make a note of what your child ate and how much he or she consumed. If you have an ingredient list, take it to the appointment. You may also make a note as to whether the food was cooked or raw. This will help your allergist rule out other conditions like Oral Allergy Syndrome or may be helpful in determining if your child may or may not consume cooked allergens such as egg or milk.

- ▶ Also note any activities you were engaging in at the time of the reaction. This might help rule out exercise-induced anaphylaxis or another condition.

- ▶ Choose a board-certified allergist-immunologist who is specifically trained to diagnose and treat food allergies. You can find allergists who are board-certified by visiting the American Board of Allergy and Immunology at www.abai.org.

COMMON FOOD ALLERGY DIAGNOSTIC TOOLS

Getting an accurate diagnosis is crucial when it comes to managing food allergies. You do not want to unnecessarily limit your child's diet or place constraints on his social interactions if you don't have to. You also do not want to miss a food allergy diagnosis and put your child at risk for having a serious allergic reaction. Once your allergist or primary care physician has taken a thorough clinical history, he or she will likely perform some form of allergy testing to confirm a suspected case of IgE-mediated food allergy.

If the clinical history is consistent with IgE-mediated food allergy, the diagnosis is typically confirmed with a skin prick test (SPT) and/or serum food-specific IgE (SpIgE).[37] If the SPT or SpIgE are negative and depending on the history, your allergist may suggest an oral food challenge to definitively diagnose or rule out food allergy.[38]

THE CLINICAL HISTORY

Getting an accurate diagnosis requires great communication skills. You have to be able to accurately convey a story and paint a picture of what is going on when you meet with your physician. As mentioned earlier, the clinical history is the most important tool for diagnosing food allergy.

In order to even begin accurately diagnosing food allergy (or any condition really), your doctor needs an accurate and complete picture of what your child has been and is experiencing. The clinical history helps to inform your physician as to which foods should be avoided, if any. It also helps the physician to consider other conditions, if any, that might be at play.

A food diary is a very helpful tool in conveying details to your physician and diagnosing food allergy, especially if you suspect multiple allergens or if it is difficult to pinpoint the suspected allergen. A food diary is also helpful when symptoms are delayed or when symptoms are more consistent with non-IgE-mediated food allergies (ex. headache, joint pain, isolated gastrointestinal symptoms).

I often suggest that mothers of children with food allergies keep an "allergic reaction journal." Keeping a daily food journal for even three days can be very cumbersome and nearly impossible for many people. An allergic reaction journal, on the other hand, is less time-consuming and more succinct. Instead of logging everything that you eat on a daily basis, I suggest that you document only suspected adverse reactions. The allergic reaction journal that I give to my clients includes a spot to note the date and time of the reaction, all foods that were eaten, what activities were taking place, symptoms observed, and any medications that were used. It is also helpful to include any pictures or ingredient labels that you may have saved. You can save these on your smart phone if you prefer digital media to paper.

SKIN PRICK TESTING (SPT)

Skin prick testing involves the introduction of minute quantities of specific allergens under the skin. The SPT is usually placed on the back or forearm. Once the skin is pricked, the allergen should be blotted off of the skin, not wiped, in order to reduce the risk of cross-contact between different allergens on the skin. After that, the waiting game begins. Each SPT site is monitored for reaction for about 10 to 20 minutes after placement. After that, any wheals are measured and compared to the control site which is typically pricked with histamine. Generally speaking, a wheal size greater than 3 mm is considered a positive result.[39] It should be noted that the skin test is a sign of sensitization and does not necessarily mean that your child is allergic to the food. This is why an accurate and detailed history is so important. If the history and skin test both suggest allergy then it is reasonable to assume an allergy diagnosis.

SPT is used to diagnose IgE-mediated food allergies only and should not be used to diagnose food-intolerances or non-IgE-mediated food allergy.[40]

ALLERGEN-SPECIFIC SERUM IGE (SPIGE)

Allergen-Specific Serum IgE (SpIgE) is a blood test that measures the level of antibodies produced in response to a specific food allergen.[41] As with SPT, a positive SpIgE test indicates sensitization to a specific food but not necessarily a clinical diagnosis of food allergy. Again this information is used in conjunction with a detailed clinical history to rule out or confirm a food allergy diagnosis.

Contrary to popular belief, the level of SpIgE does not necessarily correlate with the severity of reactions. Each allergic reaction may vary from person to person and even from time to time. You cannot predict the severity of an allergic reaction, although there are risk factors that may increase the likelihood of having a severe allergic reaction (i.e. asthma, multiple food allergies, peanut allergy, tree nut allergy, etc.). The increased concentration of food-specific IgE correlates with increased risk of clinical food allergy, not to the severity of any allergic reaction. The same is true in regards to the size of the wheals of the skin prick test. The larger size is correlated with a positive food allergy diagnosis but does not predict the severity of any future reactions.[42]

Doctors may use a combination SPT and SpIgE. Some foods may not have very good options for skin prick testing so your doctor might suggest that you bring in the actual food to be used for the SPT or test the SpIgE for that specific food.

In addition, SpIgE might be used to monitor diagnosed food allergy to see if a food allergy might be resolving.[43] A decrease in SpIgE might indicate that your child is "outgrowing" her allergy while an increase in SpIgE might suggest that a reaction is more likely to occur. It is common for allergists to retest annually to monitor food allergy diagnoses.

ORAL FOOD CHALLENGE (OFC)

Oral food challenge (OFC) is the most accurate and definitive method of diagnosing food allergy.[44] OFC involves incremental amounts of a suspected food allergen over a specific period of time.[45] An OFC should only take place in a clinical setting and under proper medical supervision so that your child can be monitored for any adverse reactions.

Double-blind placebo-controlled oral food challenge (DBPCFC) is considered the "gold standard" for diagnosing food allergy.[46, 47] In comparison to an open OFC, DBPCFC is more labor-intensive and time-consuming but it does limit bias because neither the clinician administering the test nor the patient has knowledge of when the allergen is being consumed versus the placebo. Therefore, the results are less likely to be influenced by participants.

An oral food challenge might be ordered when the clinical history and SPT or SpIgE testing is unable to confirm or exclude a food allergy diagnosis. An OFC may also be suggested before adding a food back into your child's diet when your allergist suspects that she may have "outgrown" her allergy.[48]

OTHER FOOD ALLERGY DIAGNOSTIC TOOLS

Component Resolved Diagnostics (CRD)

Component resolved diagnostics (CRD) is a type of allergy test that measures the serum IgE to individual allergen components. Foods are made up of multiple proteins and some of those proteins are, in essence, more allergenic than others. For example, in regards to testing for peanut allergy, an IgE response to the component Ara h2 is associated with a higher risk of severe allergic reaction in comparison to an IgE response to Ara h8.[49]

Recent studies have suggested that CRD may improve diagnostic accuracy and clarify potential severity of reactions. While CRD shows promise when used in conjunction with current diagnostic testing, it is not ready to replace existing allergy testing methods.[50]

Basophil Activation Test (BAT)

Basophil activation testing (BAT) is a laboratory test where the patient's basophils, a type of white blood cells, are stimulated with a particular food to determine if the cells show activation markers.

BAT is not yet commonly used in clinical settings to diagnose food allergy but growing research data suggests that BAT has higher diagnostic accuracy compared to SPT and SpIgE to peanut and to Ara h2.[51]

BAT may be useful in helping to tell the difference between children who are merely sensitized to peanut and those who are actually allergic. In addition, it may be helpful in determining the severity of reactions and might even reduce the need for oral food challenges.[52]

Elimination Diets

Elimination diets involve removing a food to see if symptoms resolve when the food is eliminated and if symptoms return when the food is added back into the diet. Elimination diets are often used to determine if a food is contributing to chronic symptoms when other testing methods are either not available or not appropriate. Elimination diets are often used to diagnose and treat non-IgE-mediated food allergies and may also be used for any adverse food reactions where symptoms are frequent or chronic.[53]

In regards to IgE-mediated food allergies, it is quite common for doctors to recommend that breast-feeding mothers follow an elimination diet if their baby is showing food allergy symptoms when the mother consumes the child's allergens. If you are breast-feeding and must eliminate certain foods from your diet, you may find it helpful to speak to a registered dietitian or nutritionist to ensure that you are getting adequate nutrition.

Food-Specific Immunoglobulin G (IgG) Testing

Food-specific IgG testing is an increasingly popular, yet controversial, method used to diagnose non-IgE-mediated food "allergies," sensitivities or intolerances. It is quite common to see it marketed straight to consumers as a way to identify a number of food hypersensitivities. In my research to learn more about IgG testing, I found a dearth of peer-reviewed articles to support its use. However, I found many journal articles, book entries, opinion letters, and position papers that state that IgG testing should not be used to identify food sensitivities, food intolerances, or food allergies.[54, 55]

The research, in fact, suggests that IgG4 actually increases with food tolerance in individuals with IgE-mediated food allergy and that the presence of IgG4 indicates the immune system is working properly.[56] The danger of someone with IgE-mediated food allergy undergoing IgG testing is that their true allergens may not show up as positive in testing. They may then think that it is safe to consume those foods based on inaccurate results. On the other hand, they may test positive for foods that they are able to tolerate. This, in turn, would further restrict an already limited diet.

I always recommend that clients first see a board-certified allergist to rule out IgE-mediated food allergy if they think they are having an adverse reaction to any foods. If you believe that your child is sensitive to wheat or gluten, you should let your primary care doctor know as soon as possible so that she can test you for Celiac disease right away. In order to get accurate test results, you must have recently consumed gluten, so do not eliminate it from your diet and then wait several months to be tested. If you do, you might get a false negative test result.

If you test negative for IgE-mediated food allergy and Celiac disease but you still feel like your child is having an adverse reaction to foods, an elimination diet, as mentioned above, is a good choice to identify food sensitivities.

AVOIDING ALLERGENS

Once your child has been diagnosed with a food allergy it is important to memorize what her food allergens are and where they hide out. Many common food allergens lurk under *scientific* names. For example, if your child is allergic to cow's milk, you need to know that casein and whey are milk proteins that must be avoided. Food allergens also hide in non-food items like hygiene products, cosmetics, cleaning supplies, craft supplies, and even bean bag chairs!

Always read ingredient lists and fabrication labels before buying or using any products. You obviously want to avoid products that contain your child's allergens as an ingredient, but you must also be cautious of products with warning labels such as: "may contain…," "processed on equipment that also processes…," or "processed in a facility that also processes…."

Label Reading

The main "treatment" for food allergy is avoiding the foods to which your child is allergic. Sounds simple enough, right? Well the first skill that you need to hone is your label reading. Let us start by discussing labeling laws so you are well-informed on what ingredient labels really mean.

FALPCA: The Good

In the United States, the Food Allergen Labeling and Consumer Protection Act of 2004 (FALPCA) requires that food manufacturers list ingredients derived from the top 8 major food allergens on the product label clearly and in plain English as opposed to using its scientific name (ex. milk vs. casein).[57] This mandate applies to domestically manufactured food products and imported pre-packaged foods.

The top 8 food allergens that are required to be listed on food ingredient labels are cow's milk, eggs, fish (e.g., bass, flounder, cod), crustacean shellfish (e.g., crab, lobster, shrimp), tree nuts (e.g., almonds, walnuts, pecans), peanuts, wheat, and soybeans. When crustacean shellfish, fish, or tree nuts are present, the specific type of shellfish, fish, or tree nut should be listed.

FALPCA: The Bad

It is important to note that FALPCA applies to pre-packaged FDA-regulated food products only, including infant formula and dietary supplements. It does not apply to raw agricultural commodities like fresh fruits and vegetables, meats, medications, alcoholic beverages or highly refined oils derived from one of the top 8 major food allergens.

Highly refined oils are not considered allergens under FALPCA because they typically have had nearly all of the allergenic protein removed and do not pose a significant risk of allergic reaction. However, all vegetable oils are required to be named under US standard food labeling laws.

While soy oil is almost always highly-refined, peanut oil may be highly-refined, expeller-pressed, or cold-pressed. Expeller-pressed and cold-pressed oils do contain allergenic proteins and could potentially trigger an allergic reaction. Because it is difficult to tell how much protein is in any given peanut oil, the safest action is to avoid it.[58]

You should also know that FALPCA does not apply to beauty or hygiene products such as cosmetics, soaps, shampoos, or lotions. This is where knowing the scientific name of your child's allergens really comes in handy. I recommend that parents make a list of the scientific names as well as common ingredients that are derived from those allergens. For instance if your child has an oat allergy, you should know that Avena Sativa is derived from oats. If your child has a coconut allergy, then you might want to look out for coconut-derived ingredients like Cocos Nucifera (coconut oil), Sodium Laurel Sulfate, Laureth-3, and many others. I like to stick with as few ingredients as possible and only buy skin products that contain familiar natural ingredients. I follow this practice with food, too, but we will get to that later.

FALPCA: The Ugly

While FALPCA is a good start, particularly if you are managing any of the top 8 major food allergies, it is severely lacking if your child has an allergy that falls outside of the top 8, such as mustard, sesame, or any other food.

We manage both mustard and sesame allergies in our household and they do present a challenge because they are often hidden under vague ingredient terms such as *natural flavor* or *spices*. If you see this on a label and your child has an allergy that falls outside of the top 8, you should either avoid giving it to your child or call the manufacturer to verify that his or her allergen is not present. Some companies will openly disclose this information and some will not. Remember, they are not required to under FALPCA.

Even if you are managing only top 8 allergies, FALPCA falls short. Contrary to popular belief, FALPCA does not proactively address the issue of cross-contact. According to the FDA, cross-contact occurs when an allergen is inadvertently introduced into a product. It is generally the result of environmental exposure during processing or handling, which may occur when multiple foods are produced in the same facility. It may occur due to use of the same processing equipment, as the result of ineffective cleaning, or from the generation of dust or aerosols containing an allergen.

A food product may be recalled if it is found to contain an undeclared allergen. It may also be removed from the market if it is mislabeled or misbranded.

Contrary to popular belief, FALPCA does not require food manufacturers to use advisory labels such as *may contain, processed in a facility that also processes,* and *processed on equipment that also processes*. These advisory statements are completely voluntary and unregulated. Because these statements are completely voluntary, you cannot assume that a product is safe just because it has no advisory statement.

In addition, you cannot judge the risk of a reaction based on the different advisory statements. A *processed in a same facility* statement is no safer than a *may contain* statement. The NAID guidelines for the diagnosis and management of food allergy suggest that products with precautionary labeling be avoided.

As food allergies increase, statements like "free from (allergens)" or "does not contain (allergens)" are becoming more common. These statements are also not regulated and sometimes can be misleading. Just a few days ago I saw a package of frozen breaded chicken tenders with the following phrases printed on the front of the box, *whole wheat, gluten free, NO wheat or gluten, NO milk or casein, NO eggs, NO peanuts or tree nuts, NO soy*. I am wondering how these whole wheat chicken tenders can be wheat free or gluten free if they contain wheat. Obviously, they can't be both whole wheat and free from wheat and gluten so this is mislabeled. This is an example of why it is so important to carefully read packaging and always read ingredient labels. Even companies that specialize in *free from* allergy-friendly food products can make mistakes or might use other allergenic ingredients outside of the top 8 allergens.

If you ever have doubt about whether or not a food is safe for your child to consume after carefully reading the ingredient label, remember you have two options. The first option is to contact the manufacturer and inquire about the ingredients, ask them about their manufacturing practices and what they do to minimize cross-contact between allergens, and be sure to have them explain their ingredient label and what any advisory labels actually mean. The other option is to simply avoid it. No food is worth risking an allergic reaction.

I would like to offer you a word of caution. Please do not let calling manufacturers take up excessive amounts of your time. Just the other day a fellow mom in the food allergy community said, "Imagine all of the free time we would have if we didn't spend so much time reading labels and calling manufacturers." Do not let this activity take time away from other things. While you will always need to read labels each and every time you buy a food product, you can greatly reduce the need to contact manufacturers if you limit the amount of prepackaged and processed foods that you buy. Whole foods are a more healthful choice and come with less risk of cross-contact. You can wash most whole foods before eating them but there's not much you personally can do to reduce the risk of cross-contact when it comes to pre-packaged foods.

AVOIDING ALLERGENS AT HOME

Many times, when I meet with the mother of a child who is newly-diagnosed with a food allergy, the first question I hear is, "Should we exclude our child's allergens from our home?" There is no right or wrong answer here. It really is a personal decision based on each family's unique situation.

Some factors to consider include your child's age, where they are developmentally, the impact on other family members' diet, whether you have the space, tools, and skills to keep allergens separate, your child's history of allergic reactions, and their individual sensitivity or threshold for reactions.

Another big factor to consider is the allergic potency of specific allergens. For example, peanuts are highly allergenic and roasting them makes them even more allergenic. On the other hand, some children with egg and milk allergies are able to tolerate baked egg or milk but cannot tolerate them in the natural form, whether raw or cooked.

Age and developmental stage is another critical factor to consider. If your child is an infant, it is unlikely that he is going to get into food that might harm him.

However, if you have a toddler who loves to explore and get into the cabinets (as many often do) she may accidentally come into contact with her allergen if precautions are not in place. Even an older child might mistakenly ingest an unsafe food if they are not trained to read labels or prevent cross-contact.

While there is no doubt that excluding your child's allergens from the home is the safest way to decrease the risk of cross-contact and an allergic reaction, it is not always possible or prudent to do so. Many families, like ours, are managing multiple children with multiple food allergies. Siblings do not always have the same allergies so completely excluding each allergen from everyone's diet would dramatically and unnecessarily limit their nutrition. We have over 15 different food allergies in our home. Some of them overlap, many of them do not. We generally exclude the allergens that overlap and occasionally use the ones that do not. The allergens that some family members can tolerate are kept separate from the other safe foods. For instance, we are completely peanut-free and nut-free but we will occasionally buy pineapple and banana, as long as they are kept separate.

My children all had cow's milk allergies as babies. Luckily, they can all tolerate it now, but they did not all gain their tolerance at the same time. At one point, we had cow's milk and two or three different milk substitutes in the house.

Color coding and using separate kitchen tools is a fantastic way to keep everyone safe. When my kids were younger they each had their own set of bowls, plates and cups so that they never mistakenly ate someone else's potentially unsafe food. This also helped me to ensure that I was serving the right meal to the right person and reduced the risk of cross-contact.

Another good practice is to use separate cooking tools to prepare meals with food allergens. For example, you might consider having a separate frying pan and spatula for frying eggs if your child has an egg allergy. In addition to pans, cutting boards, and utensils, you may consider getting separate hard-to-clean appliances and tools such as toasters, colanders, mixers, deep fryers, and waffle makers, particularly if you are managing a wheat allergy, gluten intolerance, or celiac disease.

If separate cooking tools are not an option for you, the safest practice is to make the allergy-safe food first, wash your hands, wash your kitchen supplies thoroughly with soap and water (or in the dishwasher), rinse and dry, and then make the foods that contain allergens.

In our household, most of the dishes we make are allergy-safe for every family member. Occasionally, we have to make separate batches of foods because, again, everyone does not share all of the same allergens. The goal, however, is that we are able to prepare foods that everyone can safely enjoy together.

AVOIDING ALLERGENS AWAY FROM HOME

The safest option for eating outside of the home is to bring your own food. In reality however, this is not always an option, nor is it always desirable. Being able to enjoy a meal on the go or with friends and family is an important part of socialization, but eating at restaurants or someone else's house can be a challenge if you are managing food allergies. One study surveyed 100 New York City restaurant servers and found that only 22% of them were able to correctly answer five questions about handling food allergies.[60] Many of them thought that it was safe to consume allergens in small amounts, that allergens could be destroyed by heat, and that it was okay to pick off allergens from finished dishes before serving them.[61] Despite this misinformation, over 90% of the employees reported that they felt comfortable providing a safe meal for customers with food allergies.[62] This highlights the need for us as parents of children with food allergies to communicate extensively with restaurant staff prior to eating any meal outside of the home.

When it comes to eating out with food allergies, a little planning goes a long way. Before you step into a restaurant with your crew of hungry kids, you want to do your research. Search online for allergy-friendly places to eat. It is also helpful to look up restaurant websites and review their menus. Many chains will have allergy information listed on their websites. While local restaurants might not have an allergy menu on their site, you may be able to get some idea of how accommodating they might be. Once you have a restaurant in mind, call ahead and ask them how comfortable they are with handling food allergies and what precautions they take to ensure a safe meal. If you are satisfied with their response, try to make a reservation or at least have them note your allergy and when you plan to visit the restaurant. It is usually best to choose an earlier dinner time so that the kitchen is cleaner and the staff has more time to adequately handle your meal. Remember, winging it does not work when it comes to finding a safe place to eat with food allergies. As with most things, clear communication is very important. Here are two very important topics to discuss with your server or the chef that will be handling your order.

▶ Make sure the server and kitchen staff are aware of your child's allergies. If you have more than one or two allergies, consider creating a chef's card that lists each allergen, the need to avoid these allergens or any ingredients that may contain them, and the need to avoid cross-contact.

▶ Discuss how the food is prepared so you can further reduce the risk of cross-contact. For instance, you will want to make sure that any fried foods, such as French fries, have a dedicated fryer that isn't used to fry other foods that may contain your child's allergens (ex. almond crusted-shrimp or wheat-battered chicken tenders). You want to be sure that the staff knows that your food cannot come into contact with any of your child's allergens or any tools, appliances, or surfaces that have come into contact with your child's allergens.

If the thought of all this work has you feeling overwhelmed or intimidated, that is completely understandable. Eating out with young children can be stressful. Add in food allergies and it can be downright anxiety-provoking! As I mentioned before, sometimes it can be quite a challenge to find a safe place to eat, especially if you are dealing with multiple food allergies. But eating at restaurants does have its plus side.

Eating at restaurants and other establishments is a big part of our culture and not participating in social activities that involve food can feel very isolating. So how can you and your family minimize the risk of an allergic reaction while still enjoying the opportunity to dine out once in a while? Well, here are my top tips for dining out with kids with food allergies.

- **Do your research before you go.** Search online to find restaurants that are allergy-friendly. There are websites dedicated to making your search a little easier. I particularly like the Allergy Eats mobile app. It comes in handy when traveling. Always take a look at the menu before heading out. It saves you the hassle of getting to a restaurant only to learn that there is nothing on the menu for you to eat. Always look for menus with simple dishes. I love when a restaurant has a kids' menu because those dishes are pretty simple fare. To limit the risk of cross-contact, avoid eating at places that use your particular allergens in a large number of their dishes. You will also want to avoid buffet-style restaurants and self-service food areas that are prone to cross-contact between foods, such as salad bars.

- **Call ahead.** Assuming the restaurant has some allergy-friendly dishes for you to choose, give them a ring to make sure they are accustomed to dealing with food allergies. Again, you don't want to arrive at the restaurant and find that everyone is clueless about how to safely handle food allergens and minimize cross-contact.

- **Always carry your epinephrine, other allergy medications, and your emergency plan.** This goes without saying. If you arrive at the restaurant without your allergy emergency kit, make the trip back to get it. If you have multiple children with allergies, make sure you have enough meds for each child. I have had two children have an anaphylactic reaction to the same food. You have to be prepared.

- **Make sure your table is clean.** Before you are seated, you can inform your host of your food allergies and ask that the table be cleaned, if you think it is necessary. You can also travel with your own wipes and wipe things down, as well.

If you are not comfortable with the cleanliness of your surroundings, don't be afraid to ask to have your area cleaned or to be re-seated. High chairs and booster seats are potential source of cross-contact. When my children were younger we traveled with our own booster seats and disposable placemats. You also want to avoid using the salt and pepper shakers and condiment jars on the table. They are another potential source for cross-contact. My kids have a mustard, egg, and sesame allergy so we rarely use condiments, but if you do, ask for fresh bottles or have your server bring you "to-go" packets of condiments, salt, and pepper.

▶ **Inform your server of your food allergies.** Always tell your server about your food allergies and ask to see their allergy menu, if they have one. If you can speak directly with the chef, that's great, too. Never assume a food is safe to eat without checking on the ingredients, even if you have had the same dish before and even if you already asked when you called. Make sure they understand that you or your child cannot eat food containing your allergens or that may have come into contact with your allergens.

As mentioned earlier, you might consider carrying allergy cards to give to your server. This way, they have your allergens in writing. The more ways you can communicate the better. If you feel like your server does not understand you completely or you don't feel like they can handle your food allergy requests, do not be afraid to leave. I have left restaurants that I did not think could accommodate our food allergies.

▶ **Order simple foods.** Generally speaking, it is easier to avoid "hidden" allergens by ordering simple foods with the least amount of ingredients possible or foods that don't typically have your allergen as an ingredient. The safest meal choices are whole foods such as a simply-prepared protein, vegetables, and fruits. I eat a lot of chicken breasts and veggies when I eat out. You also want to be careful about eating deep-fried items that may have come into contact with your allergens. Again, always ask your server about the safety of each dish.

▶ **Double check your order before eating.** Mistakes do happen. Even though you think you may have communicated clearly, sometimes things slip through the cracks and people make mistakes. First, when the server brings your dish, verify that it was prepared without your allergens. Second, always look at your food to make sure it does not contain any obvious allergens. I have had food prepared incorrectly on numerous occasions.

If you implement these tips you will greatly reduce the risk of having an allergic reaction and be able to enjoy dinner away from home. Remember you can live a safe, happy and healthy life with food allergies; it just takes a little extra planning.

Be sure to pass these tips onto your children, as well. Even small children can practice telling servers what their food allergies are. It is a great way to teach them how to be empowered self-advocates.

AVOIDING ALLERGENS WHILE TRAVELING

I am sure it is no surprise to you that traveling with food allergies requires a good amount of planning. There are so many choices to make such as what to pack, where to eat, where to stay, which airline to fly, what activities to do, etc. Food allergies add an additional layer of complexity to the planning process.

The Hotel

When you are thinking about booking a hotel, you want to consider how close it is to other places you might need such as a grocery store or emergency room. I always recommend staying at places that have kitchens or kitchenettes so that you can prepare your own safe meals. This is not always possible, but you can almost always request that a refrigerator and microwave be sent to your room. This way you do not have to eat out for every meal.

If your hotel has a restaurant on site, you can also call ahead to speak to the chef and check out the menu to see if it might be a suitable place for you and your family to dine. I suggest familiarizing yourself with other restaurants that are in the vicinity.

You may also want to consider shipping some safe foods to your hotel or wherever you might be staying, particularly if there aren't many grocery stores nearby.

Packing Checklist

For most people, forgetting to pack something is mostly an inconvenience. For those of us managing food allergies, forgetting to pack something can be a huge hassle and even a danger. Here are few things that you will need when traveling.

- ▶ At least two epinephrine autoinjectors per child with food allergies.

- ▶ Other medications (ex. controller inhaler, albuterol, antihistamines, etc.)

- ▶ Any medical equipment (ex. nebulizer, spacers, etc.)

- ▶ Emergency Allergy Plan

- ▶ Cell phone

- ▶ Insurance cards

- ▶ Doctors' phone numbers

- ▶ Safe snacks

- ▶ Hand wipes (in case you are unable to wash hands)

- ▶ Commercial cleaning wipes (to wipe down surfaces and airline seats)

- ▶ Make sure your child is wearing her medical alert bracelet

- ▶ Safe Toiletries (ex. allergy-safe toothpaste, lotion, bodywash, shampoo, soap, etc.)

Airplanes

Conduct a little research before you book your flight. Call a few airlines and familiarize yourself with their food allergy policies. These vary widely from airline to airline and the last thing you want is any unpleasant surprises as you are about to board the plane.

When it comes to managing food allergies, it is always safer to bring your own food. As you may have guessed, this is especially true when you are traveling on an airplane. Many airlines still serve peanuts and tree nuts on their flights and the foods that aren't actually peanuts or tree nuts usually contain them or another top 8 allergen. To say your choice of in-flight food is *limited* is an understatement. So what do you do?

When you first book your flight, either online or on the phone, you want to notify the airline of your child's peanut allergy, if she has one. Once you arrive at the airport you will also want to let the ticket agent know of your child's allergy. This will give the flight crew time to switch out the peanuts for a safer alternative if they haven't done so already. Once you arrive at your gate, you will need to notify the agent at the gate, as well. The agent will typically give you a pre-boarding pass to allow you to board the flight early so that you can clean the area around your child's seat. This is your last chance to make sure the crew is aware of your child's peanut allergy before boarding the flight.

Once you have boarded the plane, check around your child's seat for any obvious allergens and thoroughly clean the area, including the seat, seatbelt, tray table, and crevices. I recommend carrying commercial wipes as they are effective in removing allergen proteins. If you want to go one step further, you can purchase seat covers and tray table covers. You'll find a number of disposable airline seat covers and tray table covers on Amazon.com.

This goes without saying, but you need to make sure that you have your child's epinephrine, allergy and/or asthma medicines, and emergency plan with you and easily accessible. Never put your medication in a checked bag or suit case that is stowed away.

AVOIDING ALLERGENS AT SCHOOL

Avoiding allergens at school is a very important topic; one that keeps many parents up at night. In order to successfully manage food allergies at school and give everyone a little more peace of mind, children with food allergies should have an Individual Health Care Plan (IHP) that consists of a daily preventive plan and an emergency allergy plan (EAP). The emergency allergy plan outlines the exact steps that need to be taken in the case of an allergic reaction. Your allergist or pediatrician should create and go over the emergency allergy plan with you, at least annually.

The IHP is created in collaboration with you, the school nurse, your allergist, and possibly your child's principal, teacher, and other staff members. It should include daily measures to proactively reduce the risk of an allergic reaction during school, on the bus, and during any school-related functions or activities.

I highly recommend that children with food allergies also have a 504 plan in place to ensure their safety and inclusion at school. Section 504 of the Rehabilitation Act of 1973 is a federal law designed to protect the rights of individuals with disabilities in programs and activities that receive federal funding from the U.S. Department of Education.[63]

Section 504 states: "No otherwise qualified individual with a disability in the United States…shall solely, by reason of her or his disability, be excluded from the participation in, be denied the benefits of, or subjected to discrimination under any program or activity receiving federal financial assistance…".[64] Section 504 regulations require a school district to provide every child a "free appropriate public education" (FAPE) to each qualified child with a disability who is in the school's district, regardless of the nature or severity of the disability.[65]

To qualify for a 504 plan your child must be evaluated and determined to have a physical or mental impairment that substantially limits one or more major life activities. Section 504 defines a physical or mental impairment as any physiological disorder or condition, cosmetic disfigurement, or anatomical loss affecting one or more of the following body systems: neurological; musculoskeletal; special sense organs; respiratory; cardiovascular; reproductive; digestive; genito-urinary, hemic-lymphatic; skin; and endocrine; or any mental or psychological disorder.

Major life activities, under Section 504, include functions such as caring for one's self, performing manual tasks, walking, seeing, hearing, speaking, breathing, learning, and working.[66] This is not an exhaustive list of major life activities. Under the Americans with Disabilities Act Amendments of 2008 (Amendments Act), which amended the Americans with Disabilities Act of 1990 (ADA), congress outlined additional examples of major life activities including eating, sleeping, standing, lifting, bending, reading, concentrating, thinking, and communicating. Congress also provided a list of examples of "major bodily functions" that are major life activities such as the functions of the immune system, normal cell growth, digestive, bowel, bladder, neurological, brain, respiratory, circulatory, endocrine, and reproductive functions. It is important to note that this is not an exhaustive list but merely a list of examples.[67]

A life threatening food allergy impacts the immune system and limits major life activities such as eating on a daily basis. In the event of an allergic reaction, it may affect many body systems including the respiratory system, circulatory system, skin, digestive system, and of course, the immune system. An allergic reaction may also significantly limit major life activities such as breathing and eating. As we know, anaphylaxis can be fatal so it really has the potential to affect every body system and major life activity.

The first step in obtaining a 504 Plan for your child is to request a 504 evaluation to determine if your child's allergy qualifies under Section 504. The evaluation typically involves input from you, your child's pediatrician or allergist, the school nurse, the school principal, your child's teacher and other staff members who are part of the team.

It is your job to provide evidence that supports the determination that your child has a disability that qualifies under Section 504. Make sure that you have a written letter from your allergist that states that your child has a life-threatening allergy that may affect several body systems and major life activities. Your school may have paperwork for your doctor to complete, as well.

Once it is determined that your child meets the qualifications for a 504 Plan, you will work together to determine which accommodations are appropriate to ensure a safe and inclusive learning environment for your child. It is helpful to come to the 504 meeting with a list of accommodations prepared. If you have a letter from your doctor stating any necessary accommodations, that goes a long way in persuading the team to implement them.

Accommodations should cover your child's entire school day from the time they get on the school bus in the morning until they arrive back at home in the afternoon.

The 504 plan should address the following issues:

- Carrying medication on the school bus

- Training the bus driver to recognize an allergic reaction and administer epinephrine

- Rules regarding eating on the bus

- Where your child will sit on the bus (ex. assigned seat within the bus driver's view)

- Whether or not your child will self-carry epinephrine and where medications will be stored

- Who will be trained to administer epinephrine

- The need to follow the emergency allergy plan

- Will allergens be allowed in the classroom

- The cleaning protocol if eating is allowed in the classroom

- Classroom parties

- Field trips

- Projects involving food

- Rewards (ex. non-food rewards for reading logs)

- Where will your child eat lunch

- Will they be able to purchase food in the lunch room or will they pack

- ▶ Will you have safe snacks in the classroom

- ▶ After school activities

- ▶ School-wide celebrations

- ▶ Food allergy bullying

- ▶ Allowing the child to wash hands frequently

- ▶ Providing personal school supplies rather than using community school supplies

These are just some ideas of topics that you will want to address in your 504 meeting and plan. This is not an exhaustive list and some of these may not apply to your specific situation. The key is to tailor your child's 504 plan to her specific needs.

FANTASTICALLY FREE EXERCISE:

1. Make sure your allergist gives you a written list of your or your child's allergens and any foods they recommend you avoid.

2. Familiarize yourself with the common places where your child's food allergens tend to hide.

Chapter 3

KNOW WHAT TO DO DURING AN ALLERGIC REACTION

Accidents happen, so be prepared. Avoidance of known allergens is the first line of defense against having an allergic reaction. Unfortunately, accidents do happen even with a high-level of vigilance on your part.

Allergic reactions to foods can be very severe or even fatal.

Anaphylaxis is a sudden severe, life-threatening allergic reaction which can lead to constriction of the airways, drop in blood pressure, and suffocation due to swelling in the throat. During an allergic reaction, you must be able to act quickly in order to minimize the severity of the reaction, so it is very important to know what to do. You must be prepared BEFORE your child has an allergic reaction. Here are some tips to help you prepare yourself.

FOLLOW YOUR CHILD'S ALLERGY EMERGENCY PLAN

Create a Food Allergy Emergency Plan with your child's allergist (or primary care physician). Food Allergy Research and Education (FARE) has a great example of a Food Allergy Emergency Plan that you can print and give to your allergist to customize.

You can download it at: http://www.foodallergy.org/document.doc?id=234.

No matter what form you use, the emergency plan should be written out clearly and easy to understand. It should also cover the following:

- ▶ Your child's allergies

- ▶ Possible signs and symptoms of an allergic reaction

- ▶ Each action step of the allergy treatment plan and which medications should be given and when. While Epinephrine (Adrenaclick®, EpiPen®, Auvi-Q™) is the first and best response for treating anaphylaxis, your doctor may prescribe other treatments or medications (ex. Antihistamine, Albuterol, Prednisone) to be used in addition to epinephrine.

- ▶ List your contact information as well as emergency contacts.

ALWAYS CARRY TWO EPINEPHRINE AUTOINJECTORS

Always have at least two (2) epinephrine auto-injectors (and other emergency meds) with your child. Never leave home without it. Epinephrine is the only medication that treats all of the symptoms of anaphylaxis.

- ▶ Fill your epinephrine prescription immediately after it is prescribed.

- ▶ Store epinephrine at room temperature.

- ▶ Make sure you know how to use your epinephrine auto-injector. Read over the instructions and practice with the training device that comes in each package. You may also ask your doctor or nurse to demonstrate the administration with the trainer if you are still unsure or uncomfortable with using it.

- ▶ Replace any discolored or expired epinephrine auto-injectors with new ones.

- ▶ Keep an additional set of epinephrine auto-injectors at home in a designated place.

- Train your child (if age appropriate) family, friends, teachers, babysitters and anyone else who may be caring for your child on when and how to use the epinephrine auto-injector. Make sure they know where it can be found in the case of an emergency. Also, make sure they are aware of your child's Food Allergy Emergency Plan.

- Follow your child's Food Allergy Emergency Plan without hesitation. Act quickly when you notice symptoms. Administering epinephrine early on is crucial to preventing serious complications and death.

- Note that a second dose of epinephrine may be needed if your child's symptoms are not improving within 5-10 minutes of the last dose.

- Call 911 immediately after administering the first dose of epinephrine.

FANTASTICALLY FREE EXERCISE:

1. Develop a Food Allergy Emergency plan with your doctor. If you already have a plan, review it and make sure that all of the information is up-to-date.

2. Practice using your training device.

3. Make sure that everyone who cares for your child has access to your child's epinephrine auto-injectors and Food Allergy Emergency Plan.

Chapter 4

KNOW THE SIGNS AND SYMPTOMS OF AN ALLERGIC REACTION

To be fully prepared, you must know the signs and symptoms of an allergic reaction. As mentioned previously, you must be able to act fast in the event of an allergic reaction. But before you can take action, you have to be able to recognize the symptoms of an allergic reaction. Your emergency plan is useless if you do not know when you need to implement it.

If your child has a history of severe allergic reactions, administer the epinephrine auto-injector as soon as you notice symptoms of an allergic reaction. Remember, a speedy response is critical to minimizing the risk of serious complications.

Speak to your physician about the signs and symptoms of an allergic reaction. Make sure you are familiar with all of the symptoms of an allergic reaction and include them on your child's Emergency Plan. Symptoms may occur immediately after ingesting a food or may be delayed by a couple of hours. Symptoms of an allergic reaction may include:

▶ Difficulty breathing, shortness of breath, wheezing

▶ Repetitive coughing

▶ Tightness of the throat, hoarseness, swelling of the vocal chords

- ▶ Hives

- ▶ Itching of the mouth, throat, or skin

- ▶ Swelling of the tongue, lips, mouth, face, or extremities

- ▶ Lightheadedness, dizziness, fainting

- ▶ Nausea, vomiting, diarrhea

- ▶ Abdominal cramping

- ▶ Sense of impending doom, panic, anxiety

- ▶ Confusion

Be sure to discuss these and other possible symptoms with your doctor so that you feel comfortable recognizing an allergic reaction. Remember: Do not hesitate to implement your Food Allergy Emergency Plan and call 911 if you believe your child may be having a severe allergic reaction.

FANTASTICALLY FREE EXERCISE:

1. Discuss possible symptoms of an allergic reaction with your doctor and list them on your emergency action plan.

2. Explain possible symptoms to your child, family members, friends, teachers, and caregivers so they can recognize allergic reactions, as well.

Chapter 5
GET ORGANIZED

Managing food allergies takes a great deal of organization. You put your organizational skills to the test every time you go to a doctor's appointment, make a meal, hire a baby sitter, or send your child off to school. Everyday activities that used to seem simple now require a bit of planning and foresight. Managing food allergies in and of itself can take some work but once you add in the paper work, multiple food allergies or multiple children, it can be downright overwhelming if you are not organized. Fortunately, organization is a skill that can be learned and developed.

Organize an allergy emergency kit and information center. Every family that is managing food allergies should have one central location where at least one allergy emergency kit is stored along with your Food Allergy Emergency Plan. You may also want to create an allergy command center where you store allergy-related information, recipes, emergency contact information, prescriptions, etc.

Everyone in the household and anyone caring for your child within the home should be familiar with your allergy emergency kit and information center. You will also want to create an allergy emergency kit that travels with your child.

Once you and your doctor have created your food allergy emergency plan and you have filled your emergency medicine prescriptions, you can begin creating your allergy emergency kit. Your allergy emergency kit should include the following:

- ▶ All of the emergency medications your doctor has ordered (ex. Epinephrine auto-injectors, albuterol, steroids, antihistamine, etc.)

- ▶ Devices needed to deliver medications (ex. Measuring cups, measuring spoons, spacers for inhalers, etc.)

- ▶ Your Food Allergy Emergency Plan

Be sure to store your allergy emergency kit in a safe, yet convenient location. Do not lock it up or store it in a hard-to-get-to location. Make sure everyone in the house knows where it is. In addition, you may wish to create a travel emergency kit as well as additional allergy emergency kits if your child will be spending a great deal of time away from home (ex. Grandparents' house, school, daycare, camp, etc.).

FANTASTICALLY FREE EXERCISE:

1. Choose a safe and convenient place to store your emergency kit.

2. Assemble your emergency kit(s) and let everyone know where it is located.

Chapter 6

CREATE AN ALLERGY FRIENDLY ENVIRONMENT

One of my goals is to help you create a home where you and your child can relax and feel safe.

As mentioned before, the first line of defense against having a severe allergic reaction is to avoid known allergens. It is your personal decision to decide whether to exclude any or all known allergens from your home in order to make the most allergy-friendly environment as possible.

ELIMINATING FOOD ALLERGENS

Obviously, you decrease the chances of having an allergic reaction if you choose to eliminate known allergens from your home. However, you can minimize the risk by taking precautions to prevent accidental exposure and cross contact (aka cross-contamination) with known allergens.

When deciding to eliminate an allergen from the home, here are some things to consider:

- What has been the severity of past reactions? For example, has there been an anaphylactic reaction to the allergen in the past?

- How likely is cross-contact or accidental exposure to occur? For example, if you have an airborne fish allergy, you probably would NOT want to cook fish in the house. You also would NOT want to shell peanuts in the house and spread peanut dust everywhere, if you have a peanut allergy.

▶ Do you have small children in the home who might accidentally ingest the allergen or cross-contaminate surfaces with messy little fingers?

▶ Would eliminating the allergen severely limit the diet of other family members? For example, one of my daughters could drink cow's milk but not soy milk, one could drink soy milk but, not cow's milk, and one could not drink soy milk or cow's milk, and all 3 are allergic to tree nuts, so Almond milk was out of the question.

MINIMIZING CROSS-CONTACT

Managing multiple food allergies for multiple people can be tricky, but it is doable. If you choose to keep known allergens in the house, here are some tips to minimize cross-contact and accidental exposure:

▶ Everyone in the household must be accustomed to reading food labels.

▶ Everyone must know which foods are safe for whom and which foods are not safe.

▶ Discourage food sharing.

▶ Encourage everyone to wash their hands before AND after eating.

▶ Be diligent about cleaning food surfaces, refrigerators, counters, and tabletops.

▶ Quickly clean up any spilled foods.

▶ Quarantine allergens away from other foods to minimize risk of cross contact or accidental ingestions.

- Set rules regarding where foods can and cannot be eaten in the house.

- Have assigned seats at the dinner table, especially if you have young children.

- Color code dishes and utensils so that everyone knows which ones are allergy safe for them.

- Teach everyone in the home about safe food handling practices to minimize cross-contact.

REDUCING ENVIRONMENTAL ALLERGENS

It is not uncommon for those with food allergies to also have environmental allergies and/or asthma, as well. In order to create a truly allergy-friendly environment, you will want to eliminate or reduce known environmental allergens and asthma triggers, as well.

Here are some tips for reducing environmental allergens and triggers:

- Declutter and organize your space. It is hard to clean around significant amounts of clutter. Clutter easily becomes a magnet for common allergens like dust, mold, pollen, animal fur, dander, and food crumbs and residue.

- Remove, replace, and/or clean bedding, pillows, carpets, rugs, curtains, stuffed animals and other fabric items on a regular basis. They also house a lot of common allergens.

- Keep windows closed and use the air conditioning to reduce the number of airborne allergens and pollen from outside.

- Change the filter on your furnace regularly.

- Implement a weekly and even daily cleaning schedule to keep allergen exposure to a minimum.

- Use dust mite covers for pillows and mattresses.

- Choose easy to clean furnishings and avoid upholstered furniture as much as possible.

- Avoid owning pets or at least keep them out of bedrooms.

- Avoid using wood-burning fireplace or stoves which can worsen respiratory allergies. Gas-burning fireplaces are usually ok.

- Install a vented exhaust fan on your stove to reduce cooking fumes and moisture.

- Regularly clean your refrigerator to reduce mold and food spillage.

- Keep the floor free of food crumbs and take out the trash each day. This not only reduces mold and food allergens, but it also keeps insects like cockroaches (which are very allergenic) at bay.

- Make sure you have an exhaust fan in the bathroom and clean up excess moisture right away.

Taking these steps will greatly reduce the amount of allergens and asthma triggers in your home.

FANTASTICALLY FREE EXERCISE:

1. Choose a date to go through your cupboards and/or pantry and quarantine or eliminate known food allergens.

2. Create a weekly and daily household cleaning routine to reduce the number of allergens in the home.

PART II:
Living Happily

Chapter 7

ADOPT A FANTASTICALLY FREE MINDSET

You can live a safe, happy, and healthy life with food allergies! While living with food allergies does present some unique challenges, food allergies need not stop you from doing anything that you desire to do or keep you from living the life you want to live.

Research has shown that only 10% of our happiness is due to our circumstances, 50% is due to our genetic disposition, but 40% of our happiness is due to our mindset and the activities in which we wish to engage. Truly living a safe, healthy, and happy life hinges on adopting a Fantastically Free Mindset!

The Fantastically Free mindset is all about empowerment. Living Fantastically Free™ involves focusing on what you can do, not what you cannot do. Food allergies should not negatively affect your quality of life. When you adopt a Fantastically Free mindset you don't allow food allergies to impact your life negatively.

Here are 7 principles for adopting the Fantastically Free mindset:

1. **Focus on what you can eat, not on what you cannot eat.** Even people with multiple food allergies can enjoy a wide variety of foods. View your child's food allergies as your permission to explore and experiment with trying foods that you may not have tried otherwise.

2. **Focus on what you can do, not on what you cannot do.** Participate in life-giving activities that bring you and your child joy and satisfaction. Many families report a lower quality of life because they feel like they are unable to participate in activities that they enjoy. You can still do many of the things that you love to do; it just takes a little more planning.

3. **Stand steadfast.** Take unwavering responsibility for managing your child's allergies. Do whatever you feel is necessary to keep your child safe.

4. **Empower your voice and teach your child to do the same.** Be proactive, speak up about your child's food allergies, and show her how to be an empowered self-advocate.

5. **Enjoy eating a healthy diet.** Avoid unhealthy and unsafe processed foods, as much as possible. Your body and your child's body will thank you!

6. **Remain resilient.** Don't let misinformed or misguided people get you down. View it as an opportunity to educate others.

7. **Feed your spiritual appetite.** For many people managing food allergies, spirituality can be helpful in coping with the challenges of living with a life-threatening chronic condition. If you feel like this is an area that you would like to cultivate, find ways to incorporate spirituality into your daily life. It could be as simple as praying before meals or creating a meditation practice.

8. **Enjoy life! Go have fun and try to relax.** Do what you love to do and focus on the great things in your life. Keep a gratitude journal and refer to it whenever you are feeling low. It is impossible to have a negative thought and hold a sense of gratitude at the same time. Go make memories! Just remember that it might take a little extra planning (and don't forget to take your EpiPen).

FANTASTICALLY FREE EXERCISE:

1. Choose to do one fun activity every week. Write it down now and put it on your calendar.

Chapter 8

BUILD YOUR SUPPORT NETWORK

One of the things I learned when I was working in medical social work is that it takes a team to manage serious health conditions. It is no different with food allergies. A food allergy diagnosis is life-changing. It may be very overwhelming to navigate in the beginning. It is not uncommon for people to feel anxiety, grief, depression, or even isolation when they are faced with food allergies. In addition, there is so much to learn and do to stay safe. And to top it off, many people who don't deal with food allergies everyday do not understand what it takes to manage them successfully. This is can be a lot to take on by yourself, which is why it is so important to surround yourself with a team of support.

ASSEMBLE A TEAM OF SUPPORTIVE PROFESSIONALS.

Ideally, you want to have a board-certified allergist and immunologist on your team. Look for an allergist who is familiar with food allergies, not just seasonal or environmental allergies. You will also want to have a primary care physician that is knowledgeable about food allergies and supports the treatment that you and your allergist create. If you or your child also deals with other allergic issues such as eczema, you may need to add a dermatologist to your team, as well. You may also need a referral to a gastroenterologist if you have a condition such as eosinophilic esophagitis or celiac disease.

Other professionals you might want to have on your team may include:

- ▶ School nurses, teachers, and other staff that might be caring for your child.

- ▶ Dietitians and nutritionists (especially if you are dealing with multiple food allergies).

- ▶ Other professionals to help you improve your overall quality of life and well-being, such as social workers, allergy coaches, psychologists, counselors, religious leaders, etc.

Surround yourself with a supportive network of people. One of the best ways to avoid the isolation that may accompany a food allergy diagnosis is to surround yourself with others who get what you are going through.

Here are some tips for building your food allergy support network:

- ▶ Join a food allergy support group or organization. You can find local and national groups.

- ▶ Connect with other individuals who have food allergies. You can connect with people locally or through social media.

- ▶ Identify one food-allergy supportive family member or friend with whom you can share openly.

- ▶ Consider working with a food allergy coach or mentor to help you navigate the day-to-day challenges.

- ▶ Volunteer to support food allergy organizations, such as Food Allergy Research and Education (FARE) or Kids with Food Allergies.

- ▶ Attend food allergy conferences and expos.

- ▶ Take advantage of food allergy training classes and webinars.

Enlist the help of others. Be proactive in communicating the support that you need in managing your food allergies or your child's food allergies. While there are some people who *just don't get it,* there are increasingly more people who do. Never be afraid to let people know how they can help you stay safe, whether they are a server at a restaurant, your best friend, or your hometown baseball team.

The most important thing here is to get out there and connect with people who "get" food allergies and do not be afraid to share your needs with others. Not only does this help to raise awareness around food allergies, but it also goes a long way in helping you to live life to the fullest with food allergies.

FANTASTICALLY FREE EXERCISE:

1. Research adding one missing professional to your team.

2. Name one way you plan to bolster your support network.

Chapter 9

STAY SOCIALLY CONNECTED

Avoiding isolation and staying socially connected is one of the biggest challenges when it comes to living with food allergies.

Eating is such a big part of nearly every culture on the planet. We bond over food. We use food to celebrate. We mourn with food. We show gratitude with food. Nearly every holiday and social event revolves around food. Sometimes, for better or for worse, we even comfort ourselves with food when we are alone.

Given the enormous role that food plays in our lives and the emotional attachments that we as a society and as individuals have placed upon it, it is easy to see how food allergies can impact our lives, not just biologically, but socially and psychologically, as well.

SOCIAL EVENTS WITH FAMILY AND FRIENDS

Social events with family and friends can be extremely stressful if everyone is not on the same page. It is not uncommon for family members and friends to continue to serve foods that present a danger to your child after they have been diagnosed with a food allergy. In most cases, they do not do it to be mean or to exclude your child. Although sometimes folks genuinely do not care if your child is excluded, most people are willing to create a safe environment for their friends and family.

As with most situations, communication is crucial. Once your child is diagnosed with a food allergy, it makes sense to sit down with your friends and family to discuss any upcoming holidays or get-togethers. Let friends and family know ahead of time what precautions need to be taken in order to keep your child safe. Together, you can decide who will be hosting which events, where they will be held, what types of foods will be served, and what the expectations are for everyone involved. While you may not agree on every detail right away, this will give you a good start. The most important thing is to ensure your child's physical and emotional well-being.

Here are a few tips to get everyone on the same page and create a safe and fun environment for your child.

- ▶ Speak to the host ahead of time.

- ▶ Express your desire to work together to create a safe and enjoyable time for everyone.

- ▶ Make sure the host and other guests are aware of your child's allergies.

- ▶ Ask the host about menu plans and if she would like for you to bring any safe dishes to share with the other guests.

- ▶ Share ideas for safe dishes.

- ▶ If you are comfortable with the host preparing food for your child, be sure to explain to her the importance of label reading and how to avoid cross-contact.

I often recommend bringing food to any social gathering so that you know your child has something that she can safely eat. If you bring enough for everyone, then she is less likely to feel different or left out. With that being said, sometimes it's not feasible for everyone to eat exactly the same foods, especially if you are managing multiple children with multiple food allergies but the effort, when possible, is usually appreciated by everyone involved.

EATING OUT

As mentioned in Chapter 2, eating out at restaurants is a big part of socializing in our culture. I am not going to repeat everything that I said previously, but I think it is worth reiterating the importance of planning ahead before eating out. Choose allergy-friendly restaurants and, always without fail, speak to the chef and server about your child's allergies before ordering. Always confirm that a dish is free of your child's allergens before allowing him to eat. Never assume that any dish is safe for your child to eat, no matter how many times you have ordered it before.

As our children get older, we may not be the ones choosing the restaurant when it comes to social events. It is still helpful to research the restaurant ahead of time to make sure your child has safe options to eat. If there aren't any safe options, you can choose to forgo the eating and enjoy the company or contact the restaurant to see what their policy is regarding bringing in outside food. Many restaurants do not allow you to bring in outside food but they may be willing to make an exception for someone with a food allergy, especially if it is a special occasion. This option allows your child to feel included but also stay safe.

With that being said, there are restaurants that are just going to be off-limits. If you have a peanut allergy, obviously, you should not risk going into a restaurant that has peanuts strewn all over the tables and floors. You can always suggest a safer location, recommend an alternative activity, or simply decline the invitation.

PLAY DATES

Infants, toddlers, and preschoolers need social interaction with their peers, too. Often this takes place in the form of play dates. This age group presents a unique challenge in that they often do not understand the gravity of having a life-threatening food allergy and they love to explore using all of their senses. It is not uncommon for children in this age bracket to put objects in their mouth as soon as they have them in their hands. Generally speaking, the younger the child is, the more controlled the environment needs to be.

Play dates need to be free from your child's allergens. I am not a huge proponent of "blanket" food bans in general. I think you always have to look at each individual situation and circumstance when creating a safe environment for children with food allergies.

However, for this population, and especially in this situation, keeping your child's allergens out of the picture makes absolute sense. My daughter had her first anaphylactic reaction at 1 year-old when she found a miniature peanut butter cup and put it in her mouth (wrapper and all).

Here are some tips for planning a safe play date:

- ▶ Make sure the other parents are aware of your child's allergies

- ▶ Make sure they know the signs and symptoms of an allergic reaction and how and when to use epinephrine, particularly if you won't be present.

- ▶ If food is involved, make sure you know what everyone is planning to feed their child. Provide your child with a safe snack and offer to provide something for the other children, if you wish.

- ▶ Discuss the risk of cross-contact with the other children's parents.

- ▶ Offer to provide clean toys and a safe place to play to reduce the risk of an allergic reaction.

- ▶ Practice frequent hand-washing with soap and water. You can also carry hand-wipes just in case your play date takes you some place where sinks are not easily accessible.

BIRTHDAY PARTIES, SLEEPOVERS AND GET-TOGETHERS

As your child moves through the school age years, she will be invited to many social events like birthday parties, sleepovers, and a variety of get-togethers with her friends. Social gatherings with school-agers have their own set of challenges. While you don't have to worry about your child putting everything into her mouth any more, you are likely to be a bit more stressed about having less control over her environment as she ventures off without you and begins to gain some independence.

To ease your stress-level, you might consider hanging out with your child at birthday parties and other events to make sure that everything is safe for your child. It is perfectly normal for parents of children with food allergies to do this. In fact, I have found that many parents tend to stay with their younger children (ex. kindergartners and first graders) at events, whether their child has food allergies or not, so don't feel embarrassed or uncomfortable about it.

Just speak to the parent ahead of time to let them know that you will be staying for the party, if it is okay with them, of course. Most of the time, parents really appreciate having the extra help.

As your child gets older, they will likely begin doing more things on their own.

Here's what you should do to keep your child safe and ease your mind:

- ▶ Get to know your child's friends and their parents. The stronger the relationship you have with them, the more you will trust them with your child.

- ▶ Educate them on your child's allergies.

- ▶ Make sure you know what activities they will be participating in and what kinds of food will be served.

- ▶ Discuss what needs to be done to keep your child safe. Train your child's friend's parents on the signs and symptoms of an allergic reaction and when and how to use epinephrine.

- ▶ Make sure parents have a copy of your child's allergy emergency plan and your contact information.

- ► Ensure your child is carrying at least 2 epinephrine autoinjectors at all times.

- ► Be sure your child is wearing a medic alert bracelet just in case there is an emergency.

- ► Provide safe food for your child to eat.

- ► Make sure your child knows her allergies and what she can or cannot eat.

- ► Make sure your child and friend's parents know the importance of reading labels and avoiding cross-contact.

ADOLESCENTS, TEENAGERS AND YOUNG ADULTS

By the time your child has reached middle school, he should be accustomed to carrying his own epinephrine. He should also know how to administer, read labels independently, and be able to recognize symptoms of an allergic reaction. Your child is becoming more independent which means he is increasingly more responsible for managing his own food allergy. However, just like the other stages of development adolescence and young adulthood comes with its own set of challenges.

Severe and even fatal allergic reactions are more common among adolescents and young adults. Pressure to fit in and a sense of invincibility that teenagers commonly exhibit contribute to risk-taking behaviors in regards to managing their food allergies. It is not uncommon for adolescents and young adults to not always carry their epinephrine. They may even intentionally eat food that may not be safe.

At this stage it is important to reinforce safety precautions and work with your child to implement them while meeting their need for increased independence and responsibility. Research suggests that education of teenagers with food allergies and their peers (especially those they are likely to be around in social situations) might reduce risk-taking behavior and related allergic reactions.

FANTASTICALLY FREE EXERCISE:

1. Schedule one fun activity to do with family or friends.

2. Speak to your child and find out what social activities she enjoys.

Chapter 10
COMMUNICATE EFFECTIVELY WITH FRIENDS AND FAMILY

One of the most common statements I hear from mom's of children with food allergies regarding their friends and family members is, "They just don't understand." If you have been managing food allergies for any amount of time, I am sure that you have uttered the words, "They just don't get it" at some point. I know I have on several occasions.

I am amazed at how many times I have heard someone minimize the impact of food allergies. The lack of education and understanding from friends, family members, and even acquaintances can be very frustrating. Whenever anyone speaks to another person they want to feel like they have been heard and understood.

Unfortunately, it is particularly difficult for people to wrap their minds around chronic conditions like food allergies unless they have experienced them first-hand. Unlike visible disabilities, such as losing an arm or a leg, people around you have little or no reference point in regards to what might be going on inside of your child's body. They may have trouble grasping the seriousness of an allergic reaction if they have never seen someone experience anaphylaxis. It is not uncommon for people to think that mothers of children with food allergies are overreacting. This lack of awareness often leads to miscommunication and misunderstandings.

Communication breakdowns can lead to feelings of anger, anxiety, resentment, animosity, hopelessness, isolation, despair, and depression. All of these emotions negatively impact your relationships and overall quality of life. The stress brought on by conflict can also weaken your ability to take care of yourself and effectively care for your child.

Good communication fosters healthier relationships and creates an environment which supports you in managing your child's food allergies.

So how do you improve your communication skills? Let's go over a few tips for effectively communicating with family and friends who do not understand food allergies.

TELL OTHERS HOW THEY CAN HELP.

Most family members and friends really do want to help, they just don't know how. When they don't know how to help they may do annoying things like give you unsolicited advice on how to manage your condition. Instead of getting angry or frustrated with them, remember it is the thought that counts. They are trying to be helpful. In these situations, just say something like, "Thank you. I appreciate your concern. One thing I could really use your help with is XY and Z."

MANAGE EXPECTATIONS

Understand how food allergies affect the other people in your life. They are likely still clinging to the way things used to be before your child was diagnosed with a food allergy. Though it may seem insignificant compared to the adjustments you have had to make, your friends and family are also adjusting to a new way of living and relating to you. This requires a bit of patience and understanding from everyone involved.

Change can be difficult and scary. Don't be afraid to let your friends and family know what you can and cannot do. For instance, you may not be able to go to rib festival anymore but you can still enjoy the family beach vacation. Explain to them how food allergies impact you and your child but also remind them of the ways that you can connect and enjoy each other. Change is a lot easier and less frightening when we have an idea of what to expect.

SET CLEAR BOUNDARIES

Boundaries are essential to creating healthy relationships and living a healthy life in general. But they are especially important when you are living with a chronic life-threatening condition. Setting firm boundaries involves knowing your limits and communicating them to others. Get clarity around what you can and are willing to tolerate, mentally, physically, emotionally, socially, spiritually, etc. Once you have awareness of what your boundaries are you can communicate them to others and release everything that is outside of your comfort zone.

GIVE YOURSELF PERMISSION TO UPHOLD YOUR BOUNDARIES

Many women really struggle with upholding boundaries. Generally speaking, we are taught to be nurturing and polite, so many of us struggle with saying "no" and speaking up for ourselves.

When you are managing food allergies you have to be an advocate for your child and teach them how to be their own self-advocate. Do not worry about how others might react or what they might think of you. Give yourself permission to take care of your child. It is your responsibility. Remember, boundaries aren't meant to punish others, they are meant to support your well-being and the well-being of your child.

BE CLEAR, DIRECT, AND RESPECTFUL

Effective communication requires you to be clear, direct, and respectful. You can firmly uphold your boundaries without being rude. When someone has crossed one of your boundaries, calmly inform them of what your boundary is. Chances are, they were not aware of your boundary or they may have forgotten. Never assume that someone should know something if you have not told them. If you want them to know something, tell them directly.

If a friend or family member continues to cross a particular boundary, remind them of your boundary and let them know how you feel when your boundary is crossed. Also let them know the steps that you will take in order to protect your child's well-being. If they continue to cross your boundary after you have told them what your boundary is then you need to do what you must do to protect your child. In most cases, they will see that you are serious and will respect your boundary. Effective communication requires you to respect the other person, but it also requires you to respect yourself.

Follow these tips and you will see your friends and family start to come around. Be patient. It may take some people longer than others to get it. Some people may never get it and that's okay, too. Surround yourself with supportive people who do understand what you are going through and do what you need to do to create a supportive and healthy environment.

FANTASTICALLY FREE EXERCISE:

1.   Choose one communication skill to work on this week.

Chapter 11
NURTURE YOUR MARRIAGE

Dealing with any chronic condition can place a strain on any relationship. This holds true for food allergies, as well. As you are building your support network, don't forget to cultivate support at home by nurturing your marriage and strengthening your relationship with your husband, partner, or significant other.

Managing food allergies takes a considerable amount of work. You may feel like you have too little time and energy to add anything else to your plate, including quality time with your husband. However, staying connected with your husband and taking time to ensure that you both are in agreement on how you will manage food allergies will actually make your job a little bit easier and a little less stressful.

Many times mothers of children with food allergies are frustrated with their husbands because they do not feel like their husband is on the same page when it comes to managing their child's food allergies. They often complain that their husband doesn't seem to understand the serious nature of managing food allergies. Dads have been known to buy foods at the grocery store without reading the label, order pizza at a restaurant without informing the staff of their kids' allergies, or they may even forget what some of their kids' allergies are.

It's easy to see how this might be frustrating. Instead of blowing a gasket and losing your temper with your husband, try to look for ways to remedy the problem. Perhaps your husband is weak at auditory processing and would prefer to have things written down. Whatever the case may be, it is very important that the two of you approach difficult situations as partners.

If you and your husband are not on the same page, it can feel like you are managing your child's food allergies alone and that is a very heavy weight to carry by yourself.

Here are a few tips to nurture your marriage, strengthen your relationship with your husband, and turn him into your strongest food allergy ally:

EDUCATE YOUR HUSBAND ON FOOD ALLERGIES

Make sure that your husband is educated and informed about your child's food allergies. Generally speaking, it is often the mother who takes the child to their allergy appointments, so as a mother, it makes perfect sense that you would have more opportunity to learn the ins-and-outs of your child's food allergies.

Here are few things you can do to get your husband up to speed:

- ▶ **Invite your husband to come along to appointments.** If this is not possible, take notes so that you can share important information with him. You may even want to take pictures so that he has a better idea of what goes on during testing and follow-up appointments.

- ▶ **Have your husband create a list of questions that he would like to ask the doctor.** Even if he is able to attend the allergy appointments he can still express his concerns, get his questions answered, and be an active member of the team.

- ▶ **Sit down with your husband periodically** to review your child's allergies, safety precautions (like reducing the risk of exposure and carrying epinephrine), your child's medications, how to recognize an allergic reaction, and your child's emergency allergy plan.

COMMUNICATE EFFECTIVELY

As I mentioned before, good communication skills are a must when it comes to managing food allergies. Be direct with your husband so that he doesn't have to guess what you would like him to do. I know that I often expect my husband to know what I want him to do and I get upset when he doesn't figure it out on his own. Avoid that trap by telling him what you want him to do and how he can help out. Note that you may need to tell him more than once and you may need to write it down, record a message, draw a picture, or communicate it a number of different ways before he gets; we all process information in different ways. Most men do actually want to help out and be an awesome husband and father; they just need a little (or a lot of) guidance sometimes.

SPEND QUALITY TIME TOGETHER

If you are like most moms I know who have children with food allergies, you are an extremely busy woman. Not only are you busy, but you are probably a bit preoccupied with managing your child's life-threatening condition. It is completely normal to feel a bit overwhelmed in the beginning as you are learning to adapt to the changes that a food allergy diagnosis brings.

Having a supportive partner to whom you feel emotionally connected goes a long way in alleviating some of the stress and overwhelm. Staying connected and aligned with your partner takes some effort but in the long run it will help improve your quality of life and increase your ability to effectively manage your child's food allergies.

Here is what you can do to get some quality time together.

- ▶ **Schedule a date night at least once a month.** Go out and do something fun at least once a month. Don't wait for the perfect time to do it. Choose a date and stick to it.

- ▶ **Schedule some alone time together at least once a week.** You don't always have to go somewhere to spend quality time together. Block out an hour or two for you and your husband to do something without the kids around. It can be very simple, like a movie night after the kids go to bed or an early Sunday breakfast before the kids get up.

▶ **Go to sleep together.** Hugging and cuddling actually decreases anxiety so not only are you bonding with your husband, but you are also managing you own stress. Going to sleep at the same time also increases your chances of being intimate which strengthens your bond.

These are just a few tips that you can easily implement. They do not require a lot of extra time and they don't cost a lot of money. Try them out and see what a difference they make in your marriage.

FANTASTICALLY FREE EXERCISE:

1. Schedule some quality time with your husband.

Chapter 12

TAKE CARE OF YOURSELF

The need for consistent vigilance in order to prevent exposure to allergens coupled with the never-ending fear of anaphylaxis places a significant amount of stress on the parents of children with food allergies. Parents and mothers in particular, have the added stress of communicating the risks to others who are involved in caring for the child.[69] As I mentioned before, communicating to others about your child's food allergy can be very stressful and frustrating sometimes.

Unfortunately, poor quality of life is significantly more likely among parents who have more knowledge about food allergies.[70] I guess the old saying that ignorance is bliss applies in this situation; however ignorance does not help you effectively manage your child's food allergies. Parents whose children who had been to the emergency room for a food-allergy-related issue in the past year, had multiple food allergies, or where allergic to milk, eggs, or wheat also reported having a lower quality of life.

As mothers are usually the primary care-givers for children with food allergies, they typically shoulder the brunt of the stress associated with their role and experience a greater amount of anxiety compared to dads. While some level of anxiety is good for effectively managing food allergies because it motivates you to gain information and support, too much stress and anxiety can negatively impact your quality of life.[71]

In order to effectively manage your child's food allergies you have to effectively manage your own stress and take care of yourself. Doing so helps you to model positive coping skills and self-care practices.

Here are some things that you can do to take care of yourself:

- **Eat well and enjoy your food.** It is helpful for you to nourish your body and actually enjoy eating. Slow down and savor your meals. This is a lot less stressful for you and it shows your child that eating can be a fun and enjoyable experience.

- **Schedule me time.** Make an appointment with yourself at least once a month to do something that allows you to relax and reenergize.

- **Center yourself each day.** Start your day off with some quiet time to ground yourself before the stress has a chance to creep in.

- **Wind down.** Create a wind down ritual before going to bed. Engage in activities that help you relax before you go to bed. It could be something like taking a shower or warm bath, reading a book, or saying a prayer. Avoid doing things right before bed that stress you out or keep you wide awake like watching television or checking in on social media.

- **Keep a gratitude journal.** It is easy to stress about the things that are less than ideal. Instead of doing that, keep the good things top-of-mind by writing them down each day.

- **Ask for help or support when you need it.**

These are just a few ideas of ways that you can take care of yourself. The possibilities are endless. In what area of your life could you use a little bit of self-care? Make a commitment to take care of yourself. Many moms have trouble with self-care because we are so self-less when it comes to caring for our kids. It is important to remember that you can't be your best for your child if you don't take care of yourself.

FANTASTICALLY FREE EXERCISE:

1. Create a new self-care practice this week.

PART III:
Healthy Living

Chapter 13
COMMIT TO A HEALTHY MODERN LIFESTYLE

What is causing the rapid rise in food allergies? That seems to be the million dollar question these days. The simple answer is this: our modern lifestyle. It is the same thing that is causing the steep increase in every other modern chronic illness. It is our modern lifestyle.

According to Dr. Susan Prescott, we are living in an era of increased immune disease in general.[72] Over the last 50 years there has been a massive increase in the number of modern chronic illnesses including allergic diseases; autoimmune disorders like rheumatoid arthritis, multiple sclerosis, lupus, inflammatory bowel disease; and diabetes.[73] This is only a partial list.

The fact that so many of these immune diseases have increased over the same period of time is a clue that environmental changes, related to our lifestyle, are affecting our immune function.[74]

While it is clear that environmental factors are affecting the way our genes express themselves and the way that our immune system functions, it is unclear exactly which environmental factors are triggering the onset of immune diseases, in general, or food allergy, specifically. Much research is being done right now in an effort to pinpoint which environmental factors increase the risk for developing food allergy. It seems like everyone is hoping to find a smoking gun to blame for the rise in food allergy and anaphylaxis. In reality, there is not one single culprit. Most likely, there are a number of contributing factors that influence whether or not someone develops a food allergy. This makes finding a cause extremely difficult.

In the health and wellness field, we have a term called, *bio-individuality*. The concept of bio-individuality points to the fact that everyone is a unique individual and that people are affected by things differently based on their own unique make up. For example, one food may be very healthful for one person yet dangerous for another. There is no better example of this than food allergies.

This concept of bio-individuality applies to chronic illness, as well. Chronic illnesses are not acquired like genetic defects, viruses, or bacterial infections where you can pinpoint an exact cause. Chronic illnesses have a much more complex etiology. Indeed, the exact road to acquiring a chronic illness varies from person to person.

One of my mentors, Tom Malterre, author and certified nutritionist, states that all disease is caused by the interplay between an excessive amount of environmental irritants, a lack of nutrients, and genetics. An environmental irritant can be anything (ex. chemicals, stress, etc.) in the environment that adversely affects us, while nutrients can be anything (ex. vitamins, minerals, microbes, etc) that helps our bodies to function properly.

To put it simply, the modern environment in which we live causes harm by bombarding us with irritants, affects the way that our genes are expressed, and restricts the amount of good essential nutrients that we used to get just over fifty years ago.

Let us discuss some environmental factors that are believed to contribute to the development of food allergy.

EPIGENETIC CHANGES AND THE ENVIRONMENT

Food allergy is caused by a complex interplay between environmental exposures, genetic variants, gene-environment interactions and epigenetic changes.[75] Genetics alone cannot account for the massive increase in food allergy in such a short period of time. Our DNA does not change that quickly; genetic changes typically happen at an evolutionary pace. Our genes have not changed in the last fifty years but the way that they are expressed has. It is clear that epigenetic changes represent a major player in the gene-environment interaction.[76]

The prevalence of food allergy is significantly lower in developing countries, even though migrants from these countries are not protected from developing food allergies once they relocate to a developed country.[77] This suggests that the risk of food allergy greatly depends on environmental factors which are associated with the modern lifestyle.[78]

In addition, there is good evidence that immune development is under epigenetic control. Epigenetic changes determine which cytokine genes are expressed and how immature T cells will develop.[79] Evidence suggests that gene expression of these cells in newborns is influenced by maternal microbial exposure in pregnancy and that this appears to be associated with epigenetic effects.[80]

MISSING MICROBES

A diverse gut flora is considered essential to proper immune function.

The modern western lifestyle, however, limits the amount of microbes to which we are exposed. We have less childhood infections. We use more antibiotics which kill off beneficial bacteria along with the bad bacteria. We have more cesarean sections which limits the microbes that infants are exposed to during birth. Infants who are delivered vaginally have gut flora colonized by bacteria from the mother's birth canal while infants delivered by c-section have gut flora colonized by the bacteria on their mother's skin.

Though we are just beginning to understand it, the human microbiome plays a significant role in many modern chronic illnesses.

NOT ENOUGH NUTRIENTS

The Standard American Diet is woefully deficient in nutrients and extremely high in irritants like pesticides, stabilizers, emulsifiers and preservatives. It is also extremely high in sugar, salt, and unhealthy fat. Because the diet has changed so rapidly overly the last fifty years, nutritional factors are likely contributors to the rapid increase in allergic disease.[81]

While it is difficult to nail down one exact cause of the rise in food allergies, it is clear to see that the increase is associated with our modern western lifestyle. As developing countries become more industrialized, their rate of allergic disease also increases. Our modern lifestyle has benefited us in that we have less pathogenic diseases, like bacterial and viral infections, that are associated with high childhood mortality. However, we have shifted to an increase in immune diseases and other chronic illnesses. In fact, every other modern chronic illness is also associated with our modern lifestyle and many of the contributing factors overlap. The cause of chronic illness is the same, the symptoms are different.

Knowing the factors that contribute to the development of food allergies is helpful in that it allows researchers to look for ways to prevent future food allergies and hopefully, find a cure one day. While you may not be able to reverse your child's food allergies through lifestyle changes, you can make changes that support better health and decrease your child's risk of developing more modern illness down the road. Living a healthy life with food allergies requires a commitment to living a healthy modern lifestyle.

Chapter 14

SUPPORT GOOD GUT HEALTH AND BENEFICIAL MICROBES FOR A HEALTHY IMMUNE SYSTEM

About 70% of our immune system is in our gut. It is home to the largest immune network in the body.[82] It makes sense since our gut is where we interact with the outside world. Not only does our gut come into contact with many pounds of food each year but it also houses billions of bacteria. In fact, humans contain approximately 100 trillion cells but only about 10 percent of those are human cells. The rest of those are bacteria, viruses, and other microorganisms.[83]

The human microbiome is made up of all the microbes that live in and on our bodies and includes all of their genes and the metabolic capabilities they bring in supporting human health.[84] We have a symbiotic or harmonious relationship with the bacteria in our bodies. In fact, we can't live with it. We have evolved with it and it plays an important role in our overall health.

Microbes help us to digest our food, extract vitamins and minerals that we need to survive, and help our immune system to function properly. The relationship with our gut bacteria has evolved over a long period of time and is easily disrupted by changes in the modern environment.

As mentioned previously, consuming too many antibiotics, lack of exposure to microbes, and having a c-section all contribute to disrupting the human microbiome. When people hear this, they usually say something like, "Oh, my child hasn't taken that many antibiotics so that doesn't apply to me." The truth is, we get a large amount of antibiotics in our food. This includes fruits, vegetables, and animal products. It is important to buy food free from antibiotics and other chemicals that may throw off our beneficial microbial balance and contribute to the proliferation of harmful and antibacterial-resistant bacteria.

Exposure to microbes is a good thing. I used to scoff at the "hygiene theory" because I didn't consider myself excessively clean. However, today, I think that our culture as a whole is quite germaphobic. Just look at the large number of antibacterial products on the market.

Cleaner living has already altered our microbial balance.

Microbial differences are apparent in the first week of life, with infants having much lower colonization of the beneficial bacteria Lactobacillus in modernized countries.[85] These differences are linked to the increase in allergic disease as infants who go onto develop allergies also have lower levels of Bifidobacteria in the first week of life. Gut bacteria influences the development of the immune system in a number of ways. For instance, they also promote protective anti-body production and induce specialized cells to make cytokine messages that dampen the tendency for inflammation that could lead to increased gut permeability or "leaky gut." This process reduces the risk of food proteins "escaping" and triggering an allergic reaction or autoimmunity.[86] Unfortunately, for us, however, our microbiome is quite easy to disrupt.

One study found that washing dishes in the dishwasher is associated with increased risk of allergy while washing dishes by hand appeared to be protective against allergic disease. Hand-washing dishes coupled with eating fermented foods had the lowest rate of food allergy.[87] This makes sense when you consider that hand-washing dishes probably does not eliminate as many microbes as using the dishwasher and fermented foods are natural probiotics full of beneficial microbes and enzymes.

Interestingly enough, a couple of years ago, I took a fermentation class and my instructor made a point to tell us to wash our supplies by hand with soap and water. No harsh chemicals. No dishwasher. This is how it was done traditionally and she said that she wanted to keep the good bacteria alive. When it comes to food preparation, there is a lot of wisdom in doing things the way they have been done for generations; especially considering how much disease is associated with our modern lifestyle.

In the field of food allergy research, probiotics are showing some promise.

The first randomized placebo-controlled study evaluating the administration of a probiotic, Lactobacillus rhamnosus, combined with peanut oral immunotherapy found that 80% of the children were able to tolerate peanuts without any allergic symptoms for up to 5 weeks after treatment.[88] While more research is needed in this area, and you would not what to try feeding your child peanuts at home if they are allergic to them, this supports the beneficial role that microbes play in establishing tolerance to foods.

Arguably, the most important role that microbes play is helping our immune systems to function properly. Because microbes and gut health play such an important role in immunity, they affect whether or not we develop other diseases, as well.

Here are few tips for supporting good gut health and beneficial bacteria:

- **Limit your exposure to antibiotics.** Avoid foods that contain them and only take antibiotics when absolutely necessary. Antibiotics are often over-prescribed and misused for viral infections. Each time you take an antibiotic you lose beneficial bacteria. Excessive antibiotic use also contributes to the proliferation of antibiotic-resistant bacteria as other competing bacteria are killed off.

- **Abandon antibacterial products.** Good old soap and water will do. You do not need to be excessively concerned about killing every single microbe in your environment or on your skin. We need microbes to live.

- **Eat fermented foods.** Fermented foods like yogurt and sauerkraut are good source of probiotics, especially if you make your own.

▶ **Beware of antacids.** Antacid medications increase gastric pH and adversely affect the stomach's ability to break down and digest food. If food proteins are left intact, an IgE-mediated food allergy can be induced.[89]

▶ **Eat a nutrient-dense diet.** When we eat, we feed our beneficial bacteria and they help us digest our food and keep our immune system functioning properly. Eat lots of fruits and vegetables and limit the processed food. Our microbes did not evolve on a diet of processed, pre-packaged food products loaded with chemicals, pesticides, or food additives.

FANTASTICALLY FREE EXERCISE:

1. Write down two reasons why living a healthy lifestyle is important to you.

Chapter 15

MAKE GOOD NUTRITION A TOP PRIORITY

The Standard American Diet (SAD) is how we often refer to the foods that we eat in the United States and other westernized countries. It is high in processed pre-packaged foods that are often loaded with sugar, salt, fat, preservatives, emulsifiers and other additives, chemicals, pesticides, etc. It is also relatively low in fruit, vegetables, and fiber, and lacks a diversity of nutrients. The SAD is associated with increased risk of heart disease, diabetes, cancer, and almost every other modern chronic illness.

One of the silver linings of food allergies is that it forces you to read ingredients and see what is actually in your food. This can really be eye-opening. We consume a lot of food in this country that is detrimental to our health. Most people choose convenience and taste over health and nutrition. We are now paying the price with higher rates of chronic disease and whole generations of children who are dealing with a multitude of chronic conditions. One day we are going to look back on the foods that we are eating today the same way that we look at cigarettes and we are going to wonder how anyone ever thought it was a good idea.

A healthful diet is good for anyone but it is absolutely essential for children with food allergies. Because their diet is already limited by their food allergies, it is so important that they eat a nutrient-dense diet with as much diversity as possible. Every meal is important, make them all count. Children with food allergies are at risk for nutritional deficiencies which are associated with decreased school performance, delayed bone age, and increased susceptibility to infections.[90] Children with food allergies typically have heights and weights within the normal range but are often smaller for their age than children without food allergies, even when they received similar diets.[91] This suggests that children with food allergies need even greater emphasis on eating a healthful and nutrient-dense diet.

Listed below are tips to ensure that your child is eating a healthful diet that supports their health, growth, and performance.

- ▶ **Eat plenty of fresh whole foods.** Make sure your child is getting plenty of fruits and vegetables. Look for organic and antibiotic free when possible to avoid exposure to irritants that may disrupt the immune system.

- ▶ **Make sure your child is getting adequate amounts of vitamin D.** Vitamin D plays an important role in regulating the immune system and is a key player in many chronic conditions, including autoimmune disorders and possibly food allergy. Both, too little vitamin D and too much vitamin D have been associated with food allergy.[92] One way to increase your child's vitamin D level is to let him go outside to get exercise and sunshine. Our bodies need sunlight to synthesize vitamin D. Of course, you can also find vitamin D in fish, fortified products like dairy, and vitamin D supplements.

- ▶ **Eat plenty of omega-3 fats.** Dietary fats such as omega-3 fatty acids also play an important role in regulating the immune system. A decrease in consumption of omega-3 fatty acids is a possible contributing factor to the increase of food allergy.[93] You will commonly find omega-3 fatty acids in fish, fish oil, and grass-fed beef.

- ▶ **Eat a rainbow of foods.** One way to ensure that you are getting a variety of antioxidants such as vitamins C, vitamin E, selenium, carotene, and other vitamins and minerals is to eat fruits and vegetables of all different colors. Reduced antioxidant intake from fresh fruits and vegetables is believed to be a contributing factor to the rise in allergic disease by increasing susceptibility to oxidative stress and allergic inflammation.[94] If you are unable to get in a variety of foods, speak to your physician or a registered dietitian about supplementation.

▶ **Eat less prepackaged foods.** Eating less processed foods decreases your risk of cross-contact during the manufacturing process but it also decreases your exposure to harmful food additives. Food additives, particularly emulsifiers like carboxymethylcellulose (CMC) and polysorbate 80 have been found to lead to increased inflammation of the intestines.[95] This may increase the risk for metabolic disorders like diabetes, autoimmune disorders like Crohn's, and allergic disease like food allergy.

▶ **Eat more fiber.** Dietary fiber and fermentable carbohydrates act as prebiotics and promote the growth of beneficial bacteria that we need to break down our food, reduce gut permeability and reduce the risk for developing food allergies. The decrease in dietary fiber intake associated with refined modern foods is thought to be a contributing factor to inflammatory diseases of all kinds, as well as allergic diseases.[96] Many cruciferous vegetables like Brussels sprouts are high in dietary fiber.

▶ **Eat fermented foods.** Fermented foods like sauerkraut, yogurt, and kimchi, are natural probiotics. Probiotics are beneficial living microorganisms. Generally speaking, homemade fermented foods contain many more live cultures than commercial products. You can, however, purchase fermented foods from the store or buy probiotic supplements.

FANTASTICALLY FREE EXERCISE:

1. Choose one healthy food to add into your family's diet this week.

Chapter 16
LIMIT YOUR EXPOSURE TO ENVIRONMENTAL TOXICANTS AND POLLUTANTS

When looking at possible irritants that might play a role in contributing to the rise of food allergy, and modern chronic illness in general, we cannot overlook the role of environmental toxicants and pollutants.

As you may know, cigarette smoke is associated with increased risk of asthma and a number of chronic illnesses. Inhaled pollutants, such as car exhaust, are also associated with asthma. Exposure to diesel exhaust in pregnancy has been shown to affect fetal gene expression, as does cigarette smoke. This shows that environmental pollutants can modify development through epigenetic changes.[97]

There are thousands of other pollutants that we don't know much about. In the 2006 EPA Inventory Update Review Program, chemical manufacturers reported producing or importing 6,200 chemicals weighing in at 27 trillion pounds in 2005 and that's not even including fuels, pesticides, medications, or food additives.[98] Industrialization has led to many new environmental chemicals that did not exist in traditional societies.

Common sources of pollution and toxicants are skin care ingredients, pesticides, food additives, preservatives, heavy metals, air pollution, etc. These persistent organic pollutants (POPs) contaminate our air, food, and water. Some common toxicants include polychlorinated biphenyl compounds (PCBs), organochlorine pesticides, dioxins and phthalates.[99] These pollutants accumulate in our body fat over time and can increase with each generation. Many POPs have been detected in breast milk.

In regards to chemical management the American Academy of Pediatrics issued the following statement:

> "The American Academy of Pediatrics recommends that chemical management policy in the United States be revised to protect children and pregnant women and to better protect other populations. The Toxic Substance Control Act (TSCA) was passed in 1976. It is widely recognized to have been ineffective in protecting children, pregnant women, and the general population from hazardous chemicals in the marketplace. It does not take into account the special vulnerabilities of children in attempting to protect the population from chemical hazards. Its processes are so cumbersome that in its more than 30 years of existence, the TSCA has been used to regulate only 5 chemicals or chemical classes of the tens of thousands of chemicals that are in commerce. Under the TSCA, chemical companies have no responsibility to perform premarket testing or postmarket follow-up of the products that they produce; in fact, the TSCA contains disincentives for the companies to produce such data. Voluntary programs have been inadequate in resolving problems. Therefore, chemical-management policy needs to be rewritten in the United States. Manufacturers must be responsible for developing information about chemicals before marketing. The US Environmental Protection Agency must have the authority to demand additional safety data about a chemical and to limit or stop the marketing of a chemical when there is a high degree of suspicion that the chemical might be harmful to children, pregnant women, or other populations."[100]

While you may think most chemicals are safe, they actually have not undergone truly vigorous testing to prove their safety. Most testing focuses on acute symptoms, not the long-term effects of a chemical or how they might affect our health as they accumulate in our system. They also do not study chemicals in relation to how the interact together in our bodies. Chemicals are studied in isolation and for a short period of time before they go to market. Unfortunately, this is not enough to keep our children safe.

Studies suggest that many pollutants can produce epigenetic effects even at low-dose exposures.[101]

Certain POPs are known endocrine disruptors with estrogenic properties that may contribute to the rise in allergic disease, as estrogen is associated with increased severity of allergic reactions.[102]

The only way to totally eliminate your exposure to toxic chemicals and pollutants is to live in a bubble, which is not realistic. You can, however, limit your child's exposure to toxic chemicals and pollutants.

Here are some tips on how to go about it:

▶ **Eat whole foods.** Organic, when possible. Avoid crops that use pesticides and herbicides like glyphosate, also known as Roundup. Do not buy foods that list chemicals as ingredients. If you wouldn't cook with an ingredient listed on the label or you don't know what it is, don't buy it and certainly don't feed it to your child.

▶ **Ditch the plastic.** Plastics contain many harmful chemicals like phthalates and Bisphenol A (Bisphenol A). While you can find plastics that are free of these chemicals, they often contain another equally harmful chemical in its place (i.e. Bisphenol S). Glass is a much safer alternative.

▶ **Choose natural skin care products and cosmetics.** Skin care products are prone to have many harmful chemicals. You definitely want to avoid parabens, phthalates and artificial fragrances, at the very least. I recommend researching ingredients at www.ewg.org/skindeep. There you will find ratings for different ingredients and how hazardous or safe they are considered to be.

► **Stick with natural cleaning supplies whenever possible.** Avoid harsh chemical cleaners as much as possible. You can even make your own cleaning supplies with household products like vinegar, water, citrus, or essential oils.

FANTASTICALLY FREE EXERCISE:

1. Choose one area in your home and eliminate as many harmful chemicals as you can by the end of the week. When you finish that area, feel free to move on to another area.

CONCLUSION

CONGRATULATIONS ON FINISHING THIS BOOK.

You are well on your way to living Fantastically Free! If you read this entire book you are aware that managing food allergies requires a holistic approach. In other words, your approach has to take into account your child as a biological, psychological, and social being. Food allergies touch every aspect of your life. While you may not have made all of the changes suggested in the book, the most important thing about managing food allergies is finding what works for you and your child.

I would love to continue with you on your journey as you discover how to live your best life despite food allergies. If you are interested in staying connected, be sure to visit www.FantasticallyFree.com for more resources

ABOUT THE AUTHOR

Tiffany deSilva, MSW, CPC, CHC is the founder of www.FantasticallyFree.com and www.BrightFireLiving.com. Tiffany is on a mission to empower children, families, and individuals to live safe, healthy and happy lives despite food allergies.

With a background in clinical social work and healthcare; her expertise in health, wellness, and lifestyle coaching; years working in the professional organizing field; and her life experience as a mother of three children with multiple food allergies; Tiffany combines her unique skills to help families effectively manage the practical, emotional, and social aspects of living with food allergies. Tiffany understands, first-hand, that there is a big gap to bridge between being diagnosed with a food allergy and living well with it, but it can be done!

Tiffany offers one-on-one health, wellness and lifestyle coaching to mothers of children with food allergies. She also offers group classes in-person and online. In addition, she also trains other health coaches and professionals to work with families managing food allergies.

Tiffany and her work has been featured on TLC, Discovery Health, NBC, Healthful Magazine, The Columbus Dispatch, WBNS-TV, and numerous newspapers, radio shows, and other media across the United States.

If you would like Tiffany to speak to your organization, please contact her at Tiffany@BrightFireLiving.com.

REFERENCES

1   Scott A Sicherer, Hugh A Sampson, "Food Allergy." *J Allergy Clin Immunol* 117, no 2 (2006): S470-5.

2   Joshua A Boyce, et al. "Guidelines for the Diagnosis and Management of Food Allergy in the United States: Report of the NIAID-Sponsored Expert Panel." *J Allergy Clin Immunol* 126, no 6 (2010): S1-58.

3   Scott A Sicherer, Hugh A Sampson, "Food Allergy." *J Allergy Clin Immunol* 117, no 2 (2006): S470-5.

4   Janice Vickerstaff Joneja, *The Health Professionals Guide to Food Allergies and Intolerances* (Academy of Nutrition and Dietetics, 2013). 13.

5   *National Institute of Allergy and Infectious Disease.* 2010. "What is Food Allergy." Last modified November 8. http://www.niaid.gov/topics/FoodAllergy/understanding/Pages/whatIsIt.aspx.

6   *National Institute of Allergy and Infectious Disease.* 2010. "What is an Allergic Reaction to Food." Last modified December 6. http://www.niaid.nih.gov/topics/foodAllergy/understanding/Pages/allergicRxn.aspx.

7   Janice Vickerstaff Joneja, *The Health Professionals Guide to Food Allergies and Intolerances* (Academy of Nutrition and Dietetics, 2013).

8   Joshua A Boyce, et al. "Guidelines for the Diagnosis and Management of Food Allergy in the United States: Report of the NIAID-Sponsored Expert Panel." *J Allergy Clin Immunol* 126, no 6 (2010): S1-58.

9   Joshua A Boyce, et al. "Guidelines for the Diagnosis and Management of Food Allergy in the United States: Report of the NIAID-Sponsored Expert Panel." *J Allergy Clin Immunol* 126, no 6 (2010): S1-58.

10   Joshua A Boyce, et al. "Guidelines for the Diagnosis and Management of Food Allergy in the United States: Report of the NIAID-Sponsored Expert Panel." *J Allergy Clin Immunol* 126, no 6 (2010): S1-58.

[11] Tamara T Perry, A Wesley Burks, and Stacie M. Jones, "Skin Conditions Associated with Food Allergy," in Food Allergy Practical Diagnosis and Management. ed. Scott Sicherer. (Boca Raton FL: CRC Press, 2014). 71.

[12] *National Institute of Arthritis and Musculoskeletal and Skin Diseases.* 2013. "Handout on Health: Atopic Dermatitis (A type of eczema)." http://www.niams.nih.gov/ health Info/atop dermatitis/default.asp.

[13] *National Institute of Arthritis and Musculoskeletal and Skin Diseases.* 2013. "Handout on Health: Atopic Dermatitis (A type of eczema)." http://www.niams.nih.gov/ health Info/atop dermatitis/default.asp.

[14] Joshua A Boyce, et al. "Guidelines for the Diagnosis and Management of Food Allergy in the United States: Report of the NIAID-Sponsored Expert Panel." *J Allergy Clin Immunol* 126, no 6 (2010): S1-58.

[15] Joshua A Boyce, et al. "Guidelines for the Diagnosis and Management of Food Allergy in the United States: Report of the NIAID-Sponsored Expert Panel." *J Allergy Clin Immunol* 126, no 6 (2010): S1-58.

[16] Joshua A Boyce, et al. "Guidelines for the Diagnosis and Management of Food Allergy in the United States: Report of the NIAID-Sponsored Expert Panel." *J Allergy Clin Immunol* 126, no 6 (2010): S1-58.

[17] Robert G Hosey, Peter Carek, Alvin Goo, "Exercise-Induced Anaphylaxis and Urticaria." Am Fam Physician 64, no 8 (2001): 1367-1373.

[18] *National Heart, Lung, and Blood Institute.* 2014. "What is Asthma." http://www.nhlbi.nih.gov/health/health-topics/asthma#

[19] *National Heart, Lung, and Blood Institute.* 2014. "What is Asthma." http://www.nhlbi.nih.gov/health/health-topics/asthma#

[20] *National Heart, Lung, and Blood Institute.* 2014. "What is Asthma." http://www.nhlbi.nih.gov/health/health-topics/asthma#

[21] *National Heart, Lung, and Blood Institute.* 2014. "What is Asthma." http://www.nhlbi.nih.gov/health/health-topics/asthma#

[22] *American College of Asthma, Allergy and Immunology.* 2015. "Allergic Rhinitis." http://acaai.org/allergies/types/hay-fever-rhinitis

[23] John M James, Wesley Burks, Philippe A Eigenmann. *Food Allergy.* (Edinburgh: Elsevier Suanders, 2012). 81-84.

[24] John M James, Wesley Burks, Philippe A Eigenmann. *Food Allergy.* (Edinburgh: Elsevier Suanders, 2012). 84.

[25] John M James, Wesley Burks, Philippe A Eigenmann. *Food Allergy.* (Edinburgh: Elsevier Suanders, 2012). 81-84.

---

[26] KD Jackson, LD Howie, LJ Akinbami, *Trends in Allergic Conditions among Children: United States, 1997-2011*. NCHS date Brief, no 121. Hyattsville MD: National Center for Health Statistics. 2013.

[27] John M James, Wesley Burks, Philippe A Eigenmann. Food Allergy. (Edinburgh: Elsevier Suanders, 2012). 33.

[28] Ruchi Gupta, et al. "The Prevalence, Severity, and Distribution of Childhood Food Allergy in the United States." *Pediatrics* 128, no 1 (2011): e9-e17.

[29] Ruchi Gupta, et al. "The Prevalence, Severity, and Distribution of Childhood Food Allergy in the United States." *Pediatrics* 128, no 1 (2011): e9-e17.

[30] John M James, Wesley Burks, Philippe A Eigenmann. Food Allergy. (Edinburgh: Elsevier Suanders, 2012). 33.

[31] John M James, Wesley Burks, Philippe A Eigenmann. Food Allergy. (Edinburgh: Elsevier Suanders, 2012). 40.

[32] John M James, Wesley Burks, Philippe A Eigenmann. Food Allergy. (Edinburgh: Elsevier Suanders, 2012). 41.

[33] John M James, Wesley Burks, Philippe A Eigenmann. Food Allergy. (Edinburgh: Elsevier Suanders, 2012). 41.

[34] John M James, Wesley Burks, Philippe A Eigenmann. Food Allergy. (Edinburgh: Elsevier Suanders, 2012). 41.

[35] John M James, Wesley Burks, Philippe A Eigenmann. Food Allergy. (Edinburgh: Elsevier Suanders, 2012). 41.

[36] John M James, Wesley Burks, Philippe A Eigenmann. Food Allergy. (Edinburgh: Elsevier Suanders, 2012). 41.

[37] Maeve Kelleher, S. Allan Bock and Jonathan O'B Hourihane, "Diagnostic Testing," in Food Allergy Practical Diagnosis and Management. ed. Scott Sicherer. (Boca Raton FL: CRC Press, 2014). 129-164.

[38] Maeve Kelleher, S. Allan Bock and Jonathan O'B Hourihane, "Diagnostic Testing," in Food Allergy Practical Diagnosis and Management. ed. Scott Sicherer. (Boca Raton FL: CRC Press, 2014). 129-164.

[39] Maeve Kelleher, S. Allan Bock and Jonathan O'B Hourihane, "Diagnostic Testing," in Food Allergy Practical Diagnosis and Management. ed. Scott Sicherer. (Boca Raton FL: CRC Press, 2014). 129-164.

[40] Maeve Kelleher, S. Allan Bock and Jonathan O'B Hourihane, "Diagnostic Testing," in Food Allergy Practical Diagnosis and Management. ed. Scott Sicherer. (Boca Raton FL: CRC Press, 2014). 129-164.

[41] Maeve Kelleher, S. Allan Bock and Jonathan O'B Hourihane, "Diagnostic Testing," in Food Allergy Practical Diagnosis and Management. ed. Scott Sicherer. (Boca Raton FL: CRC Press, 2014). 129-164.

[42] Maeve Kelleher, S. Allan Bock and Jonathan O'B Hourihane, "Diagnostic Testing," in Food Allergy Practical Diagnosis and Management. ed. Scott Sicherer. (Boca Raton FL: CRC Press, 2014). 129-164.

[43] Maeve Kelleher, S. Allan Bock and Jonathan O'B Hourihane, "Diagnostic Testing," in Food Allergy Practical Diagnosis and Management. ed. Scott Sicherer. (Boca Raton FL: CRC Press, 2014). 129-164.

[44] Maeve Kelleher, S. Allan Bock and Jonathan O'B Hourihane, "Diagnostic Testing," in Food Allergy Practical Diagnosis and Management. ed. Scott Sicherer. (Boca Raton FL: CRC Press, 2014). 129-164.

[45] Maeve Kelleher, S. Allan Bock and Jonathan O'B Hourihane, "Diagnostic Testing," in Food Allergy Practical Diagnosis and Management. ed. Scott Sicherer. (Boca Raton FL: CRC Press, 2014). 129-164.

[46] Maeve Kelleher, S. Allan Bock and Jonathan O'B Hourihane, "Diagnostic Testing," in Food Allergy Practical Diagnosis and Management. ed. Scott Sicherer. (Boca Raton FL: CRC Press, 2014). 129-164.

[47] Jacob D Kattan and Julie Wang. "Allergen Component Testing for Food Allergy: Ready for Prime time?" *Curr Allergy Asthma Rep.* 13, no. 1 (2013): 58-63.

[48] Maeve Kelleher, S. Allan Bock and Jonathan O'B Hourihane, "Diagnostic Testing," in Food Allergy Practical Diagnosis and Management. ed. Scott Sicherer. (Boca Raton FL: CRC Press, 2014). 129-164.

[49] Jacob D Kattan and Julie Wang. "Allergen Component Testing for Food Allergy: Ready for Prime time?" *Curr Allergy Asthma Rep.* 13, no. 1 (2013): 58-63.

[50] Jacob D Kattan and Julie Wang. "Allergen Component Testing for Food Allergy: Ready for Prime time?" *Curr Allergy Asthma Rep.* 13, no. 1 (2013): 58-63.

[51] Alexandra F Santos, et al. "Basophil Activation Test Discriminates Between Allergy and Tolerance Peanut-Sensitized Children." *J Allergy Clinical Immunol.* 134, no. 3 (2014): 645-652.

[52] Alexandra F Santos, et al. "Basophil Activation Test Discriminates Between Allergy and Tolerance Peanut-Sensitized Children." *J Allergy Clinical Immunol.* 134, no. 3 (2014): 645-652.

[53] Maeve Kelleher, S. Allan Bock and Jonathan O'B Hourihane, "Diagnostic Testing," in Food Allergy Practical Diagnosis and Management. ed. Scott Sicherer. (Boca Raton FL: CRC Press, 2014). 129-164.

54 Maeve Kelleher, S. Allan Bock and Jonathan O'B Hourihane, "Diagnostic Testing," in Food Allergy Practical Diagnosis and Management. ed. Scott Sicherer. (Boca Raton FL: CRC Press, 2014). 144.

55 Steven O Stapel, et al. "Testing for IgG4 against foods is not recommended as a diagnostic tool: EAACI Task Force Report." *Allergy.* 63 (2008): 793-796.

56 Maeve Kelleher, S. Allan Bock and Jonathan O'B Hourihane, "Diagnostic Testing," in Food Allergy Practical Diagnosis and Management. ed. Scott Sicherer. (Boca Raton FL: CRC Press, 2014). 144.

57 U.S. Food and Drug Administration. "Food Allergen Labeling And Consumer Protection Act of 2004 Questions and Answers." 2005. Updated July 18, 2006. http://fda.gov/food/guidancedocumentsregulatoryinformation/allergens/ucm106890.htm

58 Marion Groetch, "Diagnostic Testing," in Food Allergy Practical Diagnosis and Management. ed. Scott Sicherer. (Boca Raton FL: CRC Press, 2014). 167

59 Joshua A Boyce, et al. "Guidelines for the Diagnosis and Management of Food Allergy in the United States: Report of the NIAID-Sponsored Expert Panel." *J Allergy Clin Immunol* 126, no 6 (2010): S1-58.

60 Jennifer S Kim, Eyal Shemesh, and Michael C Young, "Managing Food Avoidance Within the Home and Outside the Home, and Lifestyle Issues," in Food Allergy Practical Diagnosis and Management. ed. Scott Sicherer. (Boca Raton FL: CRC Press, 2014). 193.

61 Jennifer S Kim, Eyal Shemesh, and Michael C Young, "Managing Food Avoidance Within the Home and Outside the Home, and Lifestyle Issues," in Food Allergy Practical Diagnosis and Management. ed. Scott Sicherer. (Boca Raton FL: CRC Press, 2014). 193.

62 Jennifer S Kim, Eyal Shemesh, and Michael C Young, "Managing Food Avoidance Within the Home and Outside the Home, and Lifestyle Issues," in Food Allergy Practical Diagnosis and Management. ed. Scott Sicherer. (Boca Raton FL: CRC Press, 2014). 193.

63 Ed.gov. "Protecting Students with Disabilities." 2014. http://www2.ed.gov/print/about/offices/list/ocr/504faq.html

64 Ed.gov. "Protecting Students with Disabilities." 2014. http://www2.ed.gov/print/about/offices/list/ocr/504faq.html

65 Ed.gov. "Protecting Students with Disabilities." 2014. http://www2.ed.gov/print/about/offices/list/ocr/504faq.html

66 Ed.gov. "Protecting Students with Disabilities." 2014. http://www2.ed.gov/print/about/offices/list/ocr/504faq.html

67 Ed.gov. "Protecting Students with Disabilities." 2014. http://www2.ed.gov/print/about/offices/list/ocr/504faq.html

68 Margaret Sampson, Anne Munoz-Furlong, and Scott Sicherer. "Risk-Taking and Coping Strategies of Adolescents and Young Adults with Food Allergy." *Journal of Allergy and Clinical Immunology*, 117, no 6. (2006): 1440-1445.

69 Jennifer S Kim, Eyal Shemesh, and Michael C Young, "Managing Food Avoidance Within the Home and Outside the Home, and Lifestyle Issues," in Food Allergy Practical Diagnosis and Management. ed. Scott Sicherer. (Boca Raton FL: CRC Press, 2014). 203.

70 Jennifer S Kim, Eyal Shemesh, and Michael C Young, "Managing Food Avoidance Within the Home and Outside the Home, and Lifestyle Issues," in Food Allergy Practical Diagnosis and Management. ed. Scott Sicherer. (Boca Raton FL: CRC Press, 2014). 193.

71 Jennifer S Kim, Eyal Shemesh, and Michael C Young, "Managing Food Avoidance Within the Home and Outside the Home, and Lifestyle Issues," in Food Allergy Practical Diagnosis and Management. ed. Scott Sicherer. (Boca Raton FL: CRC Press, 2014). 193.

72 Susan Prescott, *The Allergy Epidemic: A Mystery of Modern Life*. (Crawley, Western Australia: UWA Publishing, 2011), 29.

73 Susan Prescott, *The Allergy Epidemic: A Mystery of Modern Life*. (Crawley, Western Australia: UWA Publishing, 2011), 29.

74 Susan Prescott, *The Allergy Epidemic: A Mystery of Modern Life*. (Crawley, Western Australia: UWA Publishing, 2011), 30.

75 Xiumel Hong and Xiaobin Wang. "Early Life Precursors, Epigenetics, and the Development of Food Allergy." *Semin Immunopathol* 34, (2012): 655-669

76 T H-Tan, et al. "The Role of Genetics and Environment in the rise of Childhood Food Allergy." Clinical & Experimental Allergy, 42, (2012): 20-29.

77 T H-Tan, et al. "The Role of Genetics and Environment in the rise of Childhood Food Allergy." *Clinical & Experimental Allergy*, 42, (2012): 20-29.

78 T H-Tan, et al. "The Role of Genetics and Environment in the rise of Childhood Food Allergy." *Clinical & Experimental Allergy*, 42, (2012): 20-29.

79 Susan Prescott, The Allergy Epidemic: A Mystery of Modern Life. (Crawley, Western Australia: UWA Publishing, 2011), 70.

80 Susan Prescott, *The Allergy Epidemic: A Mystery of Modern Life*. (Crawley, Western Australia: UWA Publishing, 2011), 30.

81 John M James, Wesley Burks, Philippe A Eigenmann. Food Allergy. (Edinburgh: Elsevier Suanders, 2012).35.

82 Susan Prescott, *The Allergy Epidemic: A Mystery of Modern Life*. (Crawley, Western Australia: UWA Publishing, 2011), 72.

[83] Rob Stein, *NPR.* "Finally a Map of All the Microbes in Your Body." June 13, 2012. http://www.npr.org/blogs/health/2012/06/13/154913334/finally-a-map-of-all-the-microbes-on-your-body.

[84] Rob Stein, *NPR.* "Finally a Map of All the Microbes in Your Body." June 13, 2012. http://www.npr.org/blogs/health/2012/06/13/154913334/finally-a-map-of-all-the-microbes-on-your-body.

[85] Susan Prescott, *The Allergy Epidemic: A Mystery of Modern Life.* (Crawley, Western Australia: UWA Publishing, 2011), 73.

[86] Susan Prescott, *The Allergy Epidemic: A Mystery of Modern Life.* (Crawley, Western Australia: UWA Publishing, 2011), 74.

[87] Anahad O' Connor. *New York Times.* "Allergy Risk May Be Tied to How You Wash Dishes." February 22, 2015. http://mobile.nytimes.com/blogs/well/2015/02/23/allergy-risk-may-be-tied-to-how-you-wash-your-dishes/

[88] Mimi L Tang, et, al. "Administration of a Probiotic with Peanut Oral Immunotherapy: A Randomized Trial." *Journal of Allergy and Clinical Immunology* 35, no. 3 (2015) 737-744. e8.

[89] Eva Untersmayr and Erika Jensen-Jarolim. "The Role of Protein Digestibility and Antacids on Food Allergy Outcomes." *Journal of Allergy and Clinical Immunology* 12, no. 6 (2008) 1301-1310.

[90] Marion Groetch, "Dietary Management" in Food Allergy Practical Diagnosis and Management. ed. Scott Sicherer. (Boca Raton FL: CRC Press, 2014). 171.

[91] Marion Groetch, "Dietary Management" in Food Allergy Practical Diagnosis and Management. ed. Scott Sicherer. (Boca Raton FL: CRC Press, 2014). 171.

[92] Xiumel Hong and Xiaobin Wang. "Early Life Precursors, Epigenetics, and the Development of Food Allergy." *Semin Immunopathol* 34, (2012): 655-669.

[93] Xiumel Hong and Xiaobin Wang. "Early Life Precursors, Epigenetics, and the Development of Food Allergy." *Semin Immunopathol* 34, (2012): 655-669.

[94] Susan Prescott, *The Allergy Epidemic: A Mystery of Modern Life.* (Crawley, Western Australia: UWA Publishing, 2011), 101.

[95] J Suez, et al. "Food Preservatives Linked to Obesity and Gut Disease." *Nature* 514 (2014): 181-186.

[96] Susan Prescott, *The Allergy Epidemic: A Mystery of Modern Life.* (Crawley, Western Australia: UWA Publishing, 2011), 103.

[97] Susan Prescott, *The Allergy Epidemic: A Mystery of Modern Life.* (Crawley, Western Australia: UWA Publishing, 2011), 105.

[98] EPA.gov. "2006 Inventory Update Reporting: Data Summary." http://www.epa.gov/oppt/cdr/pubs/2006_data_summary.pdf

[99] Susan Prescott, *The Allergy Epidemic: A Mystery of Modern Life*. (Crawley, Western Australia: UWA Publishing, 2011), 105.

[100] American Academy of Pediatrics. "Policy Statement—Chemical Management Policy Prioritizing Children's Health" Pediatrics 127, no. 5 (2011): 983-990.

[101] Susan Prescott, *The Allergy Epidemic: A Mystery of Modern Life*. (Crawley, Western Australia: UWA Publishing, 2011), 107.

[102] Susan Prescott, *The Allergy Epidemic: A Mystery of Modern Life*. (Crawley, Western Australia: UWA Publishing, 2011), 107.

www.ingramcontent.com/pod-product-compliance
Lightning Source LLC
Chambersburg PA
CBHW032115280326
41933CB00009B/845